EXTREME WEIGHT LOSS HYPNOSIS FOR WOMEN

HOW TO BURN FAT AND LOSE WEIGHT QUICKLY USING GASTRIC BAND HYPNOSIS AND GUIDED MEDITATION TECHNIQUES.

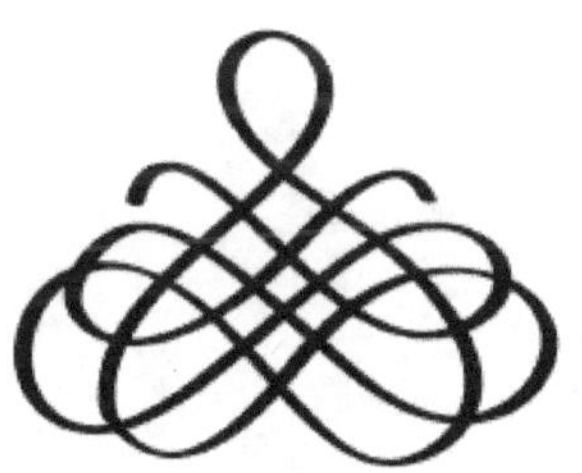

Eva Ruell

© Copyright 2020 - All rights reserved.

Table Of Contents

Introduction

Have you at any point heard how Hypnosis has helped other people reach their goals?

Maybe you have even thought about various ways you might use self-hypnosis to make changes in your own life for the better but have failed to get enough resources to do so.

The world relies on scientific evidence for almost everything. From car brakes to food hygiene, practically all safety mechanisms, from gas appliance maintenance to front door locks – rely on scientific evidence. Given that you follow the generally accepted scientific advice, you don't tend to rely on anyone's gut feeling or anecdotal evidence when it comes to the essential aspects of everyday life.

In a supersized world, people have too many options to eat and drink, but what is behind overweight is often more than the desire for a wide variety of potato chips. The diet has developed around obesity, forcing overweight people to pay a high price for expensive and risky diets, pills, or operations. Many have to cut out carbs or fats, take medications or injections, perform surgeries, or drink miracle potions. Many dieters lose weight temporarily but don't change the mindset that contributes to weight gain. The result is that after all the hard work and potentially spending thousands of dollars, most dieters regain their weight and feel even more frustrated.

The healthiest and most effective way to lose weight is not the fastest. For those who want to maintain a healthy weight and healthily lose body fat, weight loss hypnosis is what you should consider.

Weight loss should be smooth without constant hunger and constant food cravings. Weight loss hypnosis is an effective way to lose weight because it is easy to retrain your subconscious, and you can see the results immediately. Weight loss hypnosis can help you change your emotions and control your low diet.

Like all Hypnosis, weight loss hypnosis proposes weight loss while people are relaxed, as long as the suggestions correspond to what the person wants to do. Part of the focus is on changing preferences and choices for a better alimentation and to overcome appetite.

Since many dieters have negative thinking patterns that encourage them to use junk food to change their feelings, Hypnosis for weight loss also helps you see yourself as a healthy person who does not need food to change anything. You learn to see changes in eating habits not as a hardship but as empowerment because that is what you want to do in the first place.

You are getting tired. While the vast majority have the picture of the turning high contrast wheel when they consider subliminal therapy, this isn't an exact depiction. Hypnosis has been mainstream both dramatically and remedially for quite a long time and has taken on numerous structures. All the more, as of late, Hypnosis has gained decent notoriety in clinical practices for a horde of reasons. This is what you have to think about the training and why you ought to get mesmerized.

Hypnosis is a cycle of conscious mindfulness where mental portrayals supersede physiology, recognition, and conduct, referred to by numerous reliable clinical diaries. It isn't some sort of magic, and it doesn't transform you into a robot. However, it's critical to take note that entranced individuals are not dozing or oblivious. Instead, it's a hyper-mindful and hyper-responsive mental state where the brain is profoundly open to recommendations. Subsequently, an individual under Hypnosis has full concentration without doubt or ecological mindfulness.

This book contains proven steps and strategies for reprogramming your subconscious mind using self-hypnosis and unleashing the hidden power within which you have been longing.

CHAPTER 1:

What is Hypnosis for Weight Loss?

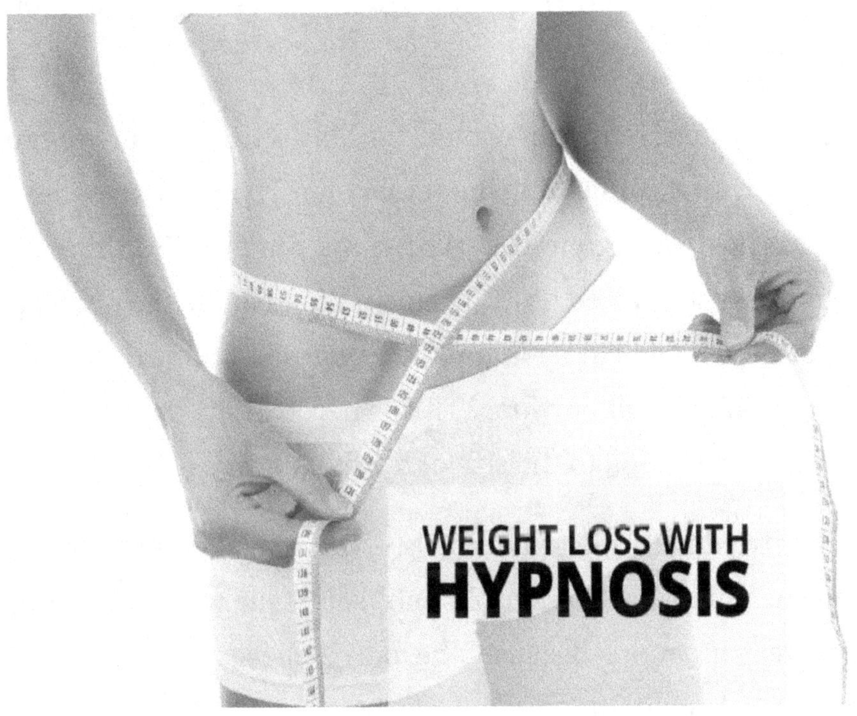

It's using hypnosis techniques to allow you to lose weight. It's a way to shed a few extra pounds. But most of the time, it is paired with a diet plan. It would help if you continued an excellent regimen of food, followed by moderate exercise. But this will allow you to lose weight faster, and if you're a person who has cravings for things, this will help you immensely.

A perfect example of this would-be Marion Corns, a woman from the United Kingdom who underwent Hypnosis to believe that she has undergone Gastric Bypass Surgery. By thinking about this, she learned how to control the amount she's eating. While she used to eat as many food plates as she wanted, she now only eats small portions. This is because she believes that her stomach shrunk to the size of a golf ball!

She has tried many diet plans before, but none of them worked as she would go back to her old habits, but she tells herself not to overeat anymore because she now believes that a gastric bypass has been done.

What's impressive, too, is the fact that she didn't undergo gastric bypass, and yet, she's able to reap the benefits. An operation would have cost her a little more than $7,000. She didn't shelve out that cash, but now, she has lost a lot of pounds—and that's all because of Hypnosis!

She underwent five sessions of gastric Hypnosis in a hospital in Spain. She was already supposed to go through the operation there, but then she found out that that the clinic also gives Gastric Hypnosis sessions, so she decided to go for that one. After five sessions, she felt like her stomach was tightening, and every time she tries to eat more than she should, she feels like she's going to throw up.

According to her, what happened was that she went through Cognitive Behavioral Therapy, which could also be a form of Hypnosis. Now, she feels like she finally fits in with society, and she no longer feels like she has to hide from people.

So how exactly does it work?

It's best to do this when you have a window of time ready for you to take care of this issue. You'll want at least thirty minutes of quiet time to handle these cravings, ideally an hour at most. You will be running some pretty heavy matters, so making sure that you're relaxed and able to return to reality before and after the Hypnosis will make it all the better.

Hypnosis works in a way that can help someone naturally feel that he is making the right choice when it comes to food. Does this mean taking away someone's willpower? It doesn't. It merely means helping someone feel better about using his will as far as food choices are concerned.

After all, losing weight is not about getting rid of something we do not want or need. People have become so focused on exercise routines and obsessed with 'healthy' foods. Of course, it is perfectly alright to pay attention to these things, but it is also important to train our brains. That is where Hypnosis comes in. Hypnosis can help in such a way that a person can create a new relationship with his body and food. Rather than taking away someone's willpower, Hypnosis can be used successfully to reinforce someone's power to choose and be more honest with these choices. For instance, you know you can always have chocolate cake, and you can have as much as you want, but do you have to have it? You know you want it, but do you need it?

There are various approaches to using Hypnosis for weight loss. Do not focus on one aspect. Choose a set of approaches relevant to that person.

Use suggestions to help the person envision the body he wants and the level of health and fitness he wants to achieve.

Use positive suggestions to help someone maximize his motivation to eat healthily.

Encourage the person to level up his fat-burning metabolism. Provide specific cues that will remind him to exercise. For instance, you can suggest that his legs will feel restless at a particular time each day, which means it is time to exercise.

Metaphors can also be used successfully. For example, you can conjure up an image in the person's mind of a sculptor facing a shapeless rock. In order to uncover the real form of that rock, the sculptor must work on it little by little, carefully and patiently. When the real form is revealed, he can get rid of the excess and needless rocks.

Another imagery you can use to help someone lose weight is to guide him into visualizing that he is wearing a fat suit. Guide him into imagining that he is able to discard layers from his fat suit. Reinforce that feeling of relief as he removes one layer at a time until the suit is in the 'right' size, the way he wants his body to look. Help the person focus not just on numbers and weight but also on health and fitness.

Help the person make a distinction between real food and fake food, the ones that are good for him and the ones that aren't.

Use a hypnotic journey metaphor. Suggest that in each step of the journey, he feels lighter and better about himself. Allow him to think about what he's wearing as he gets farther in the journey.

Use disassociation to help this person see himself in the future when he eats well, exercises regularly, looking slimmer and feeling much lighter.

Use age progression. Take him into the future where he has become slimmer. Suggest that he goes back in time from the future and remembers exactly what he needed to do to make this happen and how easy and effortless it was.

Help the person realize that when he exercises more, his will to exercise becomes greater and it becomes much easier.

Help him remember that when he feels the desire to eat unhealthily or consume food when he is not hungry, he is not reaching his goal. Let him imagine how it will make him feel to not reach his goal.

Does it Work?

The effectiveness varies from person to person. It will help you, and, on average, a person loses about six pounds. You might lose more, but you might not lose as much as expected. If you're trying to lose a ton of weight, this might not help. But, if you're looking to help eliminate cravings in your life and live a healthier lifestyle, then this is definitely the right tool for you. It's a way to help you supplement your exercising plans, and with this, you'll be able to have an even better time when it comes to shedding those pounds fast.

The Benefits

There are other benefits of using Hypnosis for weight loss. The obvious big one is that you lose weight. That's the one people will notice. You'll start to shed those pounds, and you might lose more than you expected. It won't be significant, such as like fifty pounds or more, but if you want to help your body and allow yourself the benefits of being able to control the cravings to lose weight, then this is perfect for you.

Then there are the lasting benefits of it. These are the benefits that you'll get because of the Hypnosis. When you're doing this, you'll be able to tackle those parts of your subconscious that think it's okay to eat when you're stressed, or it'll tell you to eat more than necessary. Sometimes, your mind can be your own worst enemy, and this is certainly one of those times. With Hypnosis for weight loss, you'll allow yourself to handle your body in a positive manner. If you do this, you'll actually allow yourself to control your cravings and desires through the use of Hypnosis. It might seem crazy, but it is possible.

Hypnosis for Weight Loss - What Can Hypnosis Do?

Hypnosis may be defined as a routine inducing an alternate state of awareness, which helps persons become highly sensitive to a hypnotist's suggestions.

This routine has been accepted in psychoanalysis for treating psychic illnesses by revisiting the harmful events which caused them in the past and then by transmitting suggestions created to assist them.

Hypnosis may be used to overcome phobias. Hypnosis may be used to lessen stress or tension. Hypnosis may help you remain calm before a big test and during your big speech. You will most certainly benefit from Hypnosis.

Hypnosis may regulate blood flow and different autonomic functions that are not generally subject to conscious manipulation. The relaxing reaction that occurs with Hypnosis also alters the Neuro-hormonal systems that regulate many body functions.

Hypnosis for weight loss may assist you in passing when everything else has failed. Using Hypnosis, we may aid you to achieve the weight loss that you want. Hypnosis may go straight to the middle of the matter and specialize in replacing particular behavior or habits with healthy choices.

Hypnosis may also be used to transform those who are hurt by anxiety attacks. These are characterized by the inability to concentrate, problems in making decisions, extreme sensitivity, disharmony, sleep interruptions, excessive sweating, and consistent muscle tension.

Hypnosis may aid by giving you coping systems so that you can face them in more appropriate ways whenever stress-inducing situations happen. Hypnosis may be used in many various ways.

Hypnosis may also be a method of pain control, often used with burn victims and women in labor. Hypnosis cannot depose an exercise outline but may implement and strengthen it.

Hypnotic affirmations have a cumulative therapeutic effect in the subconscious part of the mind, with the capability of improving healthy self-esteem. Hypnosis can't make a person to do anything against their will or that contradicts their values.

A Hypnotherapist has ethics that are required to create only those changes that abide by agreed-upon change work.

Hypnosis can help you obtain personal achievements and help you remain motivated toward obtaining those goals. After a few sessions of "hypnosis therapy," you may find more willingness to live and have more energy than ever imagined.

Does Weight Loss Hypnosis Work?

Mesmerizing can be thought of as an ability - a device that individuals use to unwind, change their points of view and sentiments in a more advantageous, progressively positive, and helpful way. All Hypnosis is "self-spellbinding" so the individual is 100% responsible for how it functions and the outcomes. The subliminal specialist resembles a mentor who educates and directs the individual in a loose and simple method of realizing what they need to succeed. This is totally founded on the decision to get in shape the individual makes; in any case, Hypnosis is never a substitute for an individual choice. Neither the subliminal specialist nor Hypnosis itself can "make" an individual do anything. The individual needs to get more fit.

Hypnosis is growing in popularity as a way of treating many different conditions, such as stress, smoking cessation, emotional issues, low self-esteem, fear of public speaking, and the list goes on. One of the most successful uses of Hypnosis is for weight loss. In this article, we will explore why it is gaining popularity and the reasons you should consider it for your weight control goals.

There are three specific reasons you should choose weight loss hypnosis over other weight loss programs.

Any get-healthy plan, paying little heed to what it is, expects you to be fruitful in the brain first before you can bring that accomplishment into physical reality. A decent trance specialist will educate and empower you with self-entrancing so you can generally consider yourself to be effective and stay in a positive mood concerning your weight control.

The brain looks like a muscle, and it takes exercise to get more grounded to ensure control and consistency.

Hypnosis is inexpensive in comparison to all other methods. Consider the price for gastric bypass surgery, for instance, or even special foods or diet drugs your doctor may prescribe.

The prices for some of the various weight loss programs make the fees of a hypnotist seem like nickels in comparison. Plus, you are still going to have to deal with the mind and the motivation factor. Motivation comes and goes in waves like emotions or feelings. We feel super motivated to accomplish all our goals, eat nutritious foods, work out, and improve ourselves. Then there are times you can hit an emotional wall where you feel unmotivated and dive for the first piece of chocolate or apple pie that crosses your path.

With Hypnosis, you can utilize these inner tools to develop the consistent discipline that will not only assist you to lose weight permanently but also help you take those same gifts and apply them to all other areas of your life.

CHAPTER 2:

The power of habits

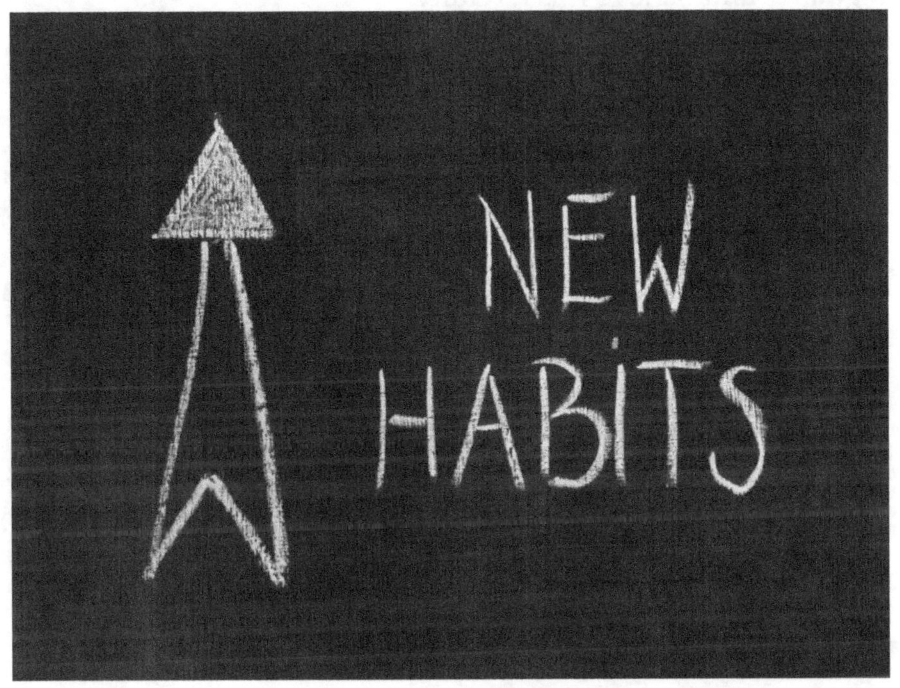

Checklist of Key Habits to Cultivate

Read through this list regularly to see if you are following these guidelines.

Visualize yourself at your ideal target weight regularly and believe it is a reality.

Repeat your affirmations daily.

Focus on your self-hypnosis techniques regularly.

Free yourself from any unpleasant habits or negative conditioning.

Do not weigh yourself or use the word diet. Do not discuss your weight with anyone. Maintain a silent, disciplined quest to improve the quality of your life.

Stick to three small, healthy major meals a day—breakfast, lunch, and dinner. Avoid eating late.

Avoid processed food and food with excess sugar, additives, or chemicals. Choose organic food when possible.

Drink fresh mineral water (that you love the taste of) between meals in place of snacking.

Always eat very slowly, chew your food thoroughly, and be fully engaged while eating. Stop eating as soon as you are full.

Be grateful for each healthy meal.

Get into the habit of moving your body as often as possible. Look for simple everyday opportunities to be active.

Exercise little and often, every day if possible, even if it is just a short walk or a mini-trampoline workout for ten minutes in the morning.

Never criticize yourself and apply the 80/20 rule.

Regularly program your mind to love your new healthy, holistic lifestyle.

Take Things Slowly

Eating should not be treated as a race. Eat slowly. This just means that you should take your time in relishing and enjoying your food, it is a healthy thing! So, how long do you have to grind up the food in your mouth? Well, there is no specific time food should be chewed, but 18-25 bites are enough to enjoy the food mindfully.

This can be hard at first, mainly if you have been used to speed eating for an exceptionally long time. Why not try some new techniques like using chopsticks when you are accustomed to spoon and fork?

Or use your non-dominant hand when eating. These strategies can slow you down and improve your awareness.

Avoid Distractions

To make things simpler for you, just make it a habit of sitting down and staying away from distractions. The handful of nuts that you eat as you walk through the kitchen and the bunch of morning snacks you nibbled while standing in front of your fridge can be hard to recall. According to researchers, people tend to eat more when they are doing other things too. You should, therefore, sit down and focus on your food to prevent mindless eating behaviors.

Savor Every Bite

Do not forget that eating mindfully is not only about enjoying the food you eat, but your health too, and without feeling guilty and uncomfortable. Relishing the sight, taste, and smell of your diet is utterly worth it. This can be so easy if you take things gradually and do not rush to perfection. Make small changes towards awareness until you are a fully mindful eater. So, eat slowly and savor the good food you are eating and the proper nutrition you give to your body.

Mind the Presentation

Regardless of how busy you are, it is good to set the table, making sure it looks divine. A lovely set of utensils, placement, and napkin made of eco-friendly cloth material is a perfect reminder that you need to sit down and pay attention when you have your meals.

Plate Your Food

Serving yourself and portioning your food before bringing the plate to the table can help you consume a modest amount, rather than putting a platter on the table from which to replenish continually. You can do this even with crackers, chips, nuts, and other snack foods.

Keep yourself away from the temptation of eating straight from a bag of chips and different types of food. It is also helpful to resize the bag or place the food in smaller containers to stay aware of the amount of food you are eating.

Having a bright idea of how much you have eaten will make you stop eating when you are full or even sooner.

Always Choose Quality over Quantity

By selecting smaller amounts of the most beautiful food within your means, you will end up enjoying and feeling satisfied without the chance of overeating.

It will be helpful if you spend time preparing your meals using quality and fresh ingredients. Cooking can be a pleasurable and relaxing experience if you only let yourself into it.

On top of this, you can achieve the peace of mind that comes from knowing what is in the food you are eating.

Do Not Invite Your Thoughts and Emotions to Dinner

Just as many other factors affect our sense of mindful eating, as well as the digestive system, it would come as no surprise that our thoughts and emotions play just as much of an important role.

It happens on the odd occasion that one comes home after a long and tiresome day and you feel somewhat "worked up," irritated and angry. This is when negative and even destructive thoughts creep in while you are having supper.

The best practice would be to avoid this altogether. Therefore, if you feel unhappy or angry in any way, go for a walk before supper, play with your children, or play with your family pet. But, whatever you do, take your mind off your negative emotions before you attempt to have a meal.

Make a Good Meal Plan for Each Week

When you start the diet, it is advised to stick to the meal plan that comes with the diet. There should be a meal plan of 2 weeks or four weeks attached to the diet's guideline. Once you are familiar with the food list, prohibited ingredients, cooking techniques, and grocery shopping for your diet, it will be easier for you to twist and change things in the meal plan. Do not try to change the meal plan for the first two weeks.

Stick to the meal plan they give you. If you try to change it right at the beginning, you may feel lost or feel terrified in the front. So, it is advised to introduce new recipes and ideas after two weeks into the diet.

Drink Lots of Water

Staying hydrated is the key to living a healthy life in general. It is not relevant for only diets, but in general, we should always be drinking enough water to keep ourselves hydrated. Dehydration can bring forth many unwanted diseases. When you are dehydrated, you feel very dizzy, lightheaded, nauseous, and lethargic. You cannot focus on anything well. Urinary infection occurs, which triggers other health issues.

Being on a diet, the purpose of drinking water is to help you process the different food you are eating and to help digest it well. Water helps in proper digestion; it helps in extracting bad minerals from our body. Water also gives us a glow on the skin.

Never Skip Breakfast

It is very essential to eat a full breakfast to keep yourself moving actively throughout the day. It gives you a significant boost, good metabolism, and your digestion starts appropriately functioning during the day. When you skip breakfast, everything sort of disrupts. Your day starts slow, and soon, you would feel restless.

It is crucial to have a good meal at the beginning of your day in order to be productive for the rest of the day.

If you are busy, try to have your breakfast on the go. Grab breakfast in a box or a mason jar and have it in the car or on the bus or whatever transport you are using to get to your work. You can also have your breakfast at a healthy restaurant where they serve food that is in sync with your diet.

Eat Protein

Protein is perfect for the body. It helps your brain function better. Protein can come from both animal and non-animal products. So even if you are a vegetable or vegan, you can still enjoy your protein from plants. Soy, mushroom, legumes, and nuts are a few examples.

Eating protein keeps you strong and healthy. Eating protein increases your brain function.

On the other hand, if you do not eat enough protein for the day, your entire way would be wasted. You will not be able to focus on anything properly. You would feel dizzy and weak all through the day. If you are a vegetarian or vegan, you can enjoy avocado, coconut, almond, cashew, soy, and mushroom to get protein.

Eat Super Foods

Most people eat foods that do not necessarily affect them in the best way. Where some foods may enhance some people's energy levels, it may impact others more negatively.

The important thing is to know your food. It may be a good idea to keep a food journal, and if you know that certain foods affect you negatively, one should try to avoid those foods and stick to healthier options.

It is a fact that most people enjoy foods which they should probably not be eating. However, if you wish to eat mindfully and enhance your health and a general sense of wellbeing, then it would be best to eat foods that will precisely do that.

There are also various foods that are classified as superfoods. These would include your lean and purest sources of protein, such as free-range chicken, as well as a variety of fresh fruit, vegetable, and herbs.

Stop Multitasking While You Eat

Multitasking is defined as the simultaneous execution of more than one activity at one time. Though it is a skill that we should master, it often leads to unproductive activity. The development of our economy leads to a more hectic way of living. Most of us develop the habit of doing one thing while doing another. This is true even when it comes to eating.

Smaller Plates, Taller Glasses

This habit changer ties in a little bit with drinking more water; however, it is a bit different. People tend to fill up their plates with food, so the size of the plate matters. If you have a large plate, you will put more food on your plate but, if you have a smaller plate, you will have less food on your plate.

Stay Positive

The secret to succeeding in anything is being optimistic. When you start something new, always stay positive regarding it. It would be best if you kept a positive mind, an open mind relatively. You cannot be anxious, hasty, and restless in a diet. You need to stay calm and do everything that calms you down. Overthinking can lead to being bored and not interested in the diet very soon. The power of positivity is immense. It cannot be compared with anything else. On the other hand, when you start something with a negative mindset, it eventually does not work out. You end up leaving it behind or failing at it because you had doubts right at the beginning. A doubtful mind cannot focus properly, and the best never comes out from a suspicious mind. Eating mindlessly can cause anyone to eat way too much, which happens to most of us. The problem is that when people are eating, they are hardly thinking about what they are doing. Instead, their minds are on other things, which leads them not to be aware of how much they are eating.

Self-discipline

What is Self-Discipline?

The term "self-discipline" is a bit of a catch-all phrase that represents a variety of different mental strengths that a person might possess. These include strengths such as restraint, perseverance, mental endurance, emotional intelligence, the ability to think before acting, the ability to finish what you started, and the strength to carry out your plans regardless of what hardships may arise on your path. When you have self-discipline, you also have self-control. You have discovered the golden ticket for avoiding unhealthy excess of anything that may lead to unwanted or negative consequences in your life, and, as a result, you find yourself achieving far greater heights of success.

Self-discipline truly is the gateway for people to move from dreaming about success to actually making success happen for themselves. When you focus on increasing your self-discipline, acting in self-disciplined ways becomes easier and easier, so, in a sense, it becomes easier for you to succeed. Now, understand that this does not mean that you will not face challenges and that your path will not be rife with hardship. You will face challenges, and things will get incredibly hard for you at various points throughout your pursuit of success. However, when you have self-discipline in your corner, arguably those challenges and hardships become less complicated because you have learned how to use your mind to help you succeed successfully. Those who have yet to increase their self-discipline find themselves using their mind against their success by allowing it to automatically come up with excuses for why they cannot create the results they desire to make in their life.

Developing self-discipline in your life does not have to be some strenuous, challenging practice that leaves you feeling like you have absolutely nothing good to look forward to. There is no reason to starve yourself from having fun, engaging in the occasional distraction, or allowing yourself to immerse yourself in your comfort zone for some time. The difference is that you are not doing these activities to stay comfortable, but instead, you are engaging in them mindfully and with the ability to stop engaging in them when you need to employ your mind for something different, such as achieving growth in any given area of your life. When you are self-disciplined, these behaviors become leisurely behaviors as they are meant to be, rather than default behaviors that prevent you from ever getting ahead in life.

Most people who pursue self-discipline agree that it is quite challenging at first, but as they begin to get the hang of it, their self-discipline becomes more enjoyable. In fact, they even start to look forward to engaging in self-discipline because it can be so fun to live a life where you are entirely in control of your actions, your impulses, and your urges, and you are capable of doing everything with great intention. Through this, you become your own most remarkable tool in your success, and, as a result, you achieve far more.

Trying to fight against your low mental toughness would be like trying to lift a 400lb weight when you have never weight trained before. It would be ludicrous to believe that you could do so consistently without seriously hurting yourself.

Likewise, there is no way that you can push against mental resistance when you lack the toughness to do so. Building your mental toughness by building your self-discipline will directly equip you with the strength you need to do all of the heavy liftings in your life and get yourself to the level of success you desire.

Why is Self-Discipline So Important?

Sure, you know that self-discipline is the number one key to success and that without it, you are going to struggle massively when it comes to achieving anything. But why is self-discipline so necessary? I mean, why can you not be successful unless you have this skill in your life?

The answer to this is simple: self-discipline is what is going to directly drive you through any challenge or setback you face in your life, especially on the path to achieving your goals.

The power of faith

Are you determined to lose weight? You want to prevent heart disease complications, diabetes, and elevated cholesterol levels associated with being overweight for most individuals, including yourself. However, because of their fitness, not everyone goes on a quest to lose weight. You can want to lose weight because you see weight loss as a way to make others look desirable and improve your self-image. To recover your usual body weight, there are several preventive steps you might take. People worldwide spend thousands and even millions of dollars annually on losing weight by attempting these steps. Exercise gadgets, healthier organic foods, dietary supplements, slimming pills, diets, and fitness clubs are spent on these vast amounts of money every day.

That simple little secret of weight loss is the magic response. You must change the way you think about yourself and your food. Take this case: do you recall those times, when you were on that expensive wonder diet, that you watched your weight rigorously but still struggled to keep your eyes off that creamy dessert after meals or didn't even feel bold enough to cut off your chocolate craving?

It may not be as easy for you to believe, but I can assure you that the reason you feel you're losing the war is easy. The explanation is that you have not changed the habits of your old thoughts about how you felt about the creamy dessert and the chocolate bar and, more importantly, about yourself. This example is to show you that your thinking patterns can influence your weight loss.

As human beings, our emotions and beliefs affect our actions, which then cause us to respond in a certain way to a situation. The little thoughts you used to have about the beautiful dessert or chocolate after your meals would have prompted you to choose to skip the dessert or just take a bite and then finish it all. Unfortunately, your above intervention will be to the detriment of your effort at losing any weight.

You may also regulate your emotions, on the other hand, or make suggestions in your mind to alter how you feel about the dessert and chocolate. The good news is that you can control your emotions or make suggestions to your mind on how you react to the dessert or the pudding without weakening your weight loss program. Hypnosis will show you how you can make these suggestions to control the emotions in the head.

Hypnosis is an interaction between yourself and the hypnotist. A hypnotist is someone who is trained to use hypnotic methods or therapy and is skilled. The hypnotist will attempt to manipulate or make suggestions on your thoughts and behavior during this interaction by specifically focusing on ideas and images that may elicit any expected results verbally.

You can receive advice from the hypnotist to lose weight through Hypnosis that will change your previous emotions or perceptions about the factors that could have contributed to your weight gain. You may also opt not to see the hypnotist face to face when you chose to use Hypnosis.

In addition to this being the overview of the mechanism of helping to facilitate progress, it also happens to be a mechanism that many of us have found works naturally. Some of us have come upon the process of programming our minds with our ambitions and accomplishments, and milestones we aspire to and have been able to proceed and accomplish them.

CHAPTER 3:

Reprogram your mind

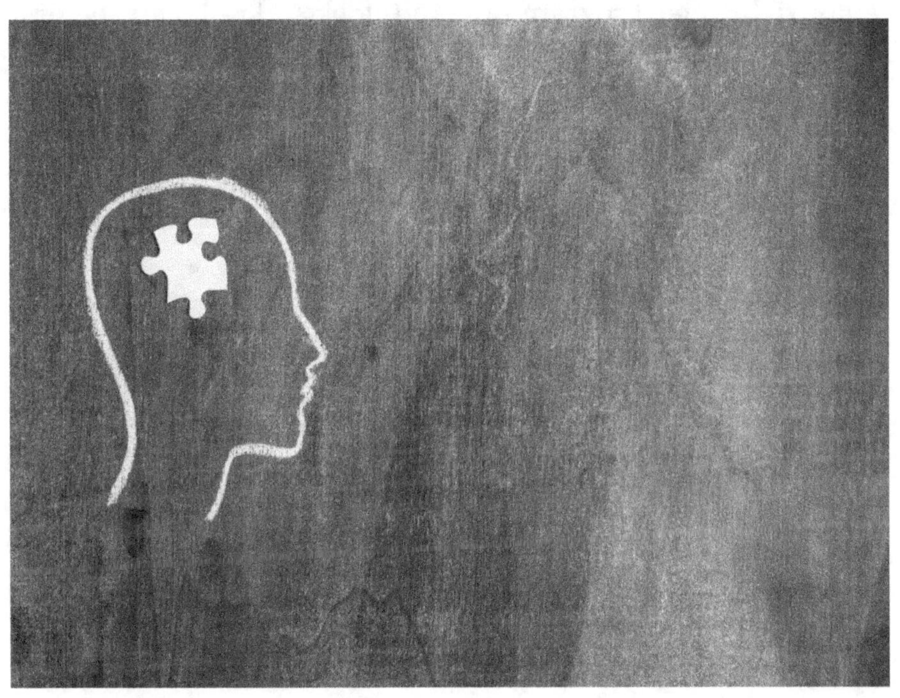

o you remember the first time you learned to do something new, for example, drive a new car? You may have driven for years but learning all about an unfamiliar vehicle can be frustrating. How do you turn on the lights or the windshield wipers? Is the gas tank filled from the left or right side? Programming the clock and radio for the first time can take a while. The first trip or two can be difficult. But then you learn where everything is and how it all works, and the mechanics become almost an automatic, unconscious process.

You can use that same inherent learning ability to teach yourself to love exercising and healthy food. You can learn to love feeling fit and healthy and to find fattening food repulsive. Whatever your weight loss aims, you can reprogram your mind in specific ways to help you achieve your goals. Learning these new habits is a matter of repetition.

The more you visualize and absorb these affirmations, the quicker you create the new inner belief. It is also gratifying because you will create very relaxing mental states that benefit your general health and well-being.

How Affirmations Work

A goal is a specific target that you set for yourself to achieve within a fixed time frame. An affirmation is a statement of intent that you repeat to yourself repeatedly. Affirmations need to be phrases and phrases said clearly and concisely with a slight emphasis. Whenever you use your claims, feel as though you are drawing the words inside you, as though you are teaching the inner part of yourself a new belief. You must always state affirmations in the present tense and focus on them as if they are a reality now. You must decide the wording of your affirmations upon before you begin a self-hypnosis session, and you must work on only one goal at a time. For example, don't work on releasing fear and losing weight in the same session. While you can use several affirmations in one session, they must all relate to the one chosen goal for that session. You must make affirmations completely unambiguous and always accentuate the positive. I use the words "I love to ..." to start many of my affirmations because love is a useful, emotive phrase, and I find this confirmation has a profound impact.

Writing your goals and affirmations is very important because it gives words power and meaning, reminding you constantly of where you are heading. It also spells out your intent loud and clear, adding clarity to your aims and helping to compound your new belief structures.

Bringing Yourself Back to Full Consciousness

If you practice this process before going to sleep, you need not count up from one to ten. Before you begin your consultation, just tell yourself that the trance will become a deep, natural sleep from which you may wake within the morning feeling nice and refreshed.

Think of the analogy of reprogramming a computer with new data. What you put into it will come back out. Totally immerse yourself in your aims. When you are in a trance, use all of your senses to compound the phrases and make your affirmations and visualizations colorful and real. Do not worry if you are not good at visualizing; you may have a different dominant sense. Most people are visual, but others absorb information more easily through another sense—feeling, hearing, smell, or even taste. That is why it is vital to use all of your senses when visualizing so that your more dominant understanding will help you absorb the new beliefs at a deeper level.

The Power of Your Mind

Never underestimate the power you have inside you. Your mind has incredible potential. All around the world, there are stories of human beings achieving impossible feats. There are documented instances of moms being able to summon superhuman strength to lift a vehicle off the floor to keep their youngsters trapped underneath.

When the mother sees her baby in a hazard, she doesn't prevent and think; I can't elevate that vehicle because it weighs too much. The handiest concept in her thoughts is to save her toddler; the truth that the car is too heavy to raise does not enter her thinking. This is the vital thing to how she will do it—there isn't a doubt in her mind, and she is entirely focused on lifting the automobile. Through excessive awareness and sheer force of will, the mom can summon the electricity to boost an automobile weighing greater than a ton.

The survival instinct is the most effective driver humans possess, and while this is threatened, in extreme circumstances, we can do matters that defy logic. When we're at serious risk, our focus turns heightened, and we enter an altered country of consciousness. In this modified nation, we can use exceptional strength and electricity.

By using self-hypnosis, you may engage your thoughts similarly and reap so much. Think of the tale of the mom lifting the automobile as a metaphor for your fitness journey. Never put a limit on what you may do. You can reap, in reality, something while you discover ways to the awareness of your thoughts.

CHAPTER 4:

The importance of having goals

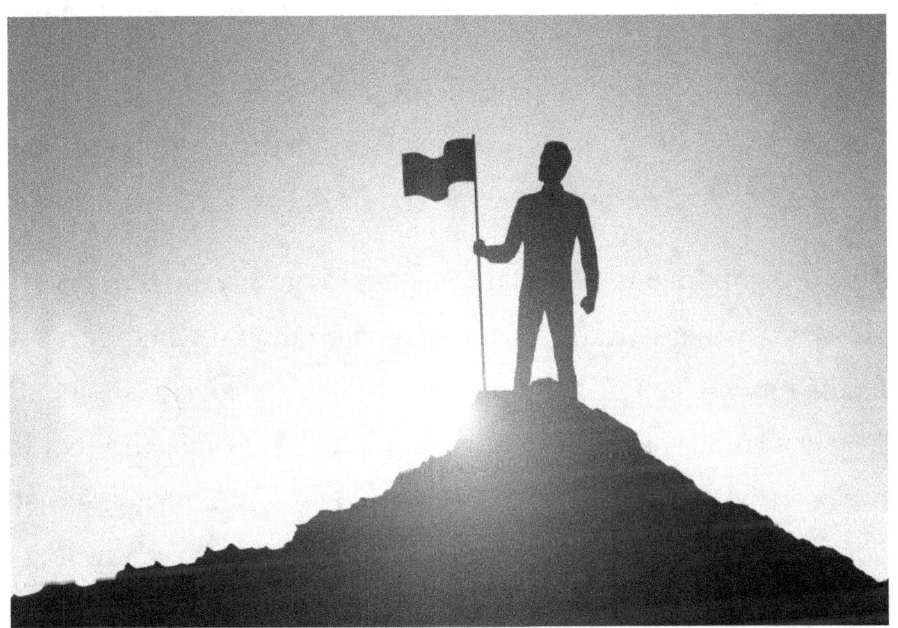

It's a good idea to grab a food journal to track you're eating on a day-to-day basis, so you are practicing awareness of what you are eating. This helps you consciously process what you are about to put into your mouth or reflect on what you already ate on any given day. It's been shown that when you are more conscious of your choices, you make better ones.

It is essential to be realistic about your goals, and you must discuss this with your surgeon. I also need to note here; for some individuals, the BMI chart can be deceiving.

This does not mean you get a free pass to bypass the BMI chart. However, it's essential to see where you fall and whether it's a factor in your actual body fat percentage overall. As someone who is 5'11 tall, I know I'm never going to be 160lbs, and that is precisely what the chart shows I should be. I'm not saying that you should hide your head in the sand or state you're 'big-boned' if you're not.

The goal is for you to lose weight and to be healthy for your body's height. It's all about proportion. The goal here is NOT to get you down to a specific weight per se, but to get you to a weight that YOU are comfortable at, and at a weight and size in which you feel good living in your body. You, feeling comfortable in your own body, makes all the difference.

Let's look at your personal goals for the short-term and long-term to help you understand where you want to be.

What are the realistic goals for your weight and height?

How much do you expect to lose overall?

What is your height?

What was your highest weight?

What was your Surgery Weight?

What is your Current Weight?

What is your ideal ending Goal Weight?

What are your post-surgery (pounds lost) goals for:

Month 1:

What size do you want to be in?

How do you want to feel?

Month 3:

What size do you want to be in?

How do you want to feel?

Month 6:

What size do you want to be in?

How do you want to feel?

Month 9:

What size do you want to be in?

How do you want to feel?

Month 12:

What size do you want to be in?

How do you want to feel?

Month 18:

What size do you want to be in?

How do you want to feel?

Month 24:

What size do you want to be in?

How do you want to feel?

Month 30:

What size do you want to be in?

How do you want to feel?

Month 36:

What size do you want to be in?

How do you want to feel?

If you don't know what you want, how will you go after it?

Clarity is so important. Knowing what you want is step one. If you do not yet know what you will do once you lose the weight, start thinking about it now.

The plan is to lose weight and to do all the things you have not had the opportunity to do as an obese individual. There's so much more life for you to live and many things I know you want to do.

Do you have a desire to travel to Europe and walk through the ancient streets of Rome?

Do you want to walk/run a 5k?

Do you want to chase after your grandchildren and be able to pick them up at a moment's notice?

Or would you like to feel comfortable making love to your husband/wife?

What is it that means the most to you?

What are those things that you're excited to do now that you're losing weight?

List them out.

CHAPTER 5:

Step-by-Step Hypnotherapy for Weight Loss

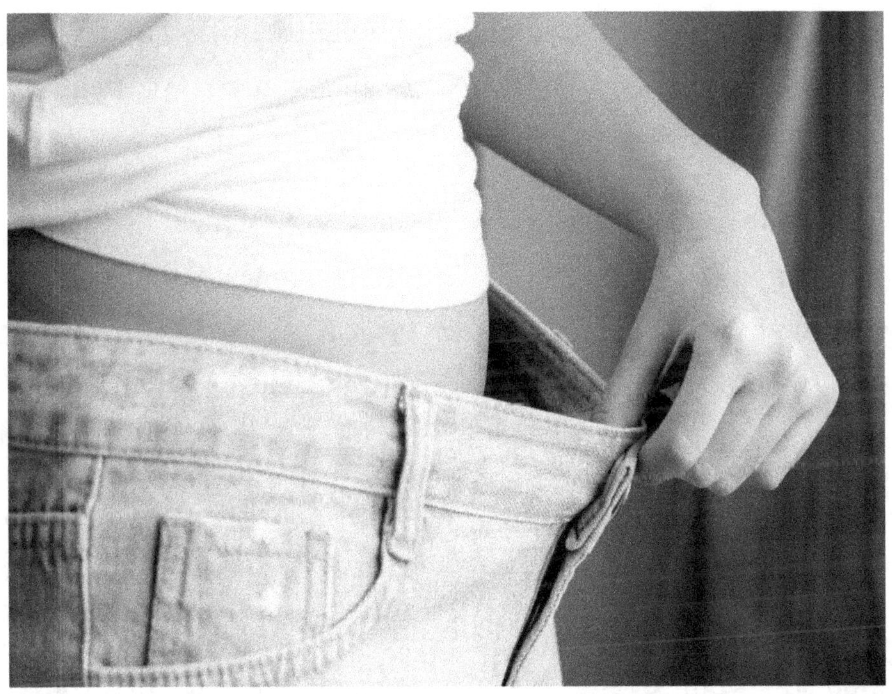

If you don't figure entrancing will enable you to change your emotions, it will probably have little impact.

Become agreeable. Go to a spot where you may not be stressed. This can resemble your bed, a couch, or a pleasant, comfortable chair anyplace. Ensure you bolster your head and neck. Wear loose garments and ensure the temperature is set at an agreeable level. It might be simpler to unwind if you play some delicate music while mesmerizing yourself, particularly something instrumental.

Focus on an item. Discover something to take a gander at and focus on in the room, ideally something somewhat above you. Utilize your concentration for clearing your leader of all contemplations on this item. Make this article the main thing that you know about.

Breathing is crucial. When you close your eyes, inhale profoundly. Reveal to yourself the greatness of your eyelids and let them fall delicately. Inhale profoundly with an ordinary mood as your eyes close. Concentrate on your breathing, enabling it to assume control over your whole personality, much like the item you've been taking a gander at previously. Feel progressively loose with each fresh breath. Envision that your muscles disperse all the pressure and stress. Permit this inclination from your face, your chest, your arms, lastly, your legs to descend your body.

When you're entirely loose, your psyche should be clear, and you will be a self-mesmerizing piece.

Display a pendulum. Customarily, the development of a pendulum moving to and from has been utilized to energize the center is spellbinding. Picture this pendulum in your psyche, driving to and from. Concentrate on it as you unwind to help clear your brain.

Start by focusing on 10 to 1 in your mind. You advise yourself as you check down that you are steadily getting further into entrancing. State, "10, I'm alleviating. 9, I get increasingly loose. 8. I can feel my body spreading, unwinding. 7, Nothing yet unwinding I can handle.... 1, I'm resting profoundly. Keep in mind that you will be in a condition of spellbinding when you accomplish one all through.

Waking up from self-hypnosis. Once during spellbinding, you have accomplished what you need, you should wake up. From 1 to 10, check back. State in your mind: "1, I wake up. 2, I'll feel like I woke up from a significant rest when I tally down. 3, I feel wakeful more.... 10, I'm wakeful, I'm new.

Develop a plan. Reinventing your mind with spellbinding requires consistent redundancy. You ought to endeavor in a condition of spellbinding to go through around twenty minutes per day. While beneath, shift back and forth between portions of the underneath referenced methodologies. Attempt to assault your poor eating rehearses from any edge.

Learn to refrain from emotional overeating. One of the main things you should endeavor to do under mesmerizing is to influence yourself. You are not intrigued by the frightful nibble of food you experience issues kicking. Pick something that you will, in general, revel in, like frozen yogurt. State, "Dessert tastes poor and makes me feel debilitated." Repeat twenty minutes until you're prepared to wake up from the trance. Keep in mind; excellent eating regimen doesn't suggest you have to quit eating; simply eat less awful sustenance. Simply influence yourself to devour less food, you know, is undesirable.

Write your very own positive mantra. Self-spellbinding ought to likewise be utilized to reinforce your longing to eat better. Compose a mantra to rehash in a trance state. It harms me and my body when I overeat.

Imagine the best thing for you. Picture what you might want to be more beneficial to support your longing to live better. From when you were more slender, take a picture of yourself or do your most extreme to figure what you'd resemble in the wake of shedding pounds. Concentrate on this image under mesmerizing. Envision the trust you'd feel on the off chance that you'd be more advantageous. This will cause you to comprehend that when you wake up. Eat each supper with protein. Protein is especially valuable at topping you off and can improve your digestion since it advances muscle improvement. Fish, lean meat, eggs, yogurt, nuts, and beans are great wellsprings of protein. A steak each dinner might be counterproductive, yet in case you're eager, eating on nuts could go far to helping you accomplish your objectives.

Eat a few modest meals daily. If you don't eat for quite a while, your digestion will go down, and you will stop fat consumption. If you expend something modest once every three or four hours, your metabolism will go up, and when you plunk down for dinner, you will be less hungry.

Eat organically grown foods. You will be loaded up with foods grown from the ground and furnish you with supplements without putting any pounds on. To start shedding pounds, nibble on bananas rather than treats to quicken weight reduction.

Cut down on unhealthy fats. It tends to be helpful for you to have unsaturated fats, similar to those in olive oil. Nonetheless, you should endeavor to limit your saturated fat and trans-fat intake. Both of these are significant factors that add to coronary illness.

Learn more about healthy cooking. In preparing meals, trans fats are common, mainly when eating meals, sweets, and fast food.

Saturated fats may not be as bad as trans fats. However, they might be undesirable. Primary saturated fat sources include spreads, cheddar cheese, grease, red meat, and milk. The journey to weight loss is not an easy one. A person needs a lot of help and motivation to succeed. With the use of hypnotherapy, one can easily stay the course and watch the pounds melt away. Following the guide above and with a credible hypnotherapist or mastering self-hypnosis will help you achieve your goals.

The Benefits of Hypnotherapy for Losing Weight

Hypnotherapy that is geared towards helping you lose weight can help you develop a more positive image. The session usually starts with accepting your situation and doing something about it, not because of the pressure of society but because of health reasons.

Hypnosis will reframe your mind and will help you better understand you're "why" or the reason behind your goal for weight loss. This alternative session will help you manage your weight because it directly taps your motives and self-interest.

Another benefit of hypnotherapy for weight loss is it can help you relieve stress. The meditative component of Hypnosis can help you achieve a calmer and more relaxed mind. Relieving stress is important in weight loss as studies show the connection between stress and an increase in appetite.

Hypnotherapy will also rewire your conscious and subconscious mind so you can feel good about exercise and healthy diets. These two components go hand in hand in weight loss, and through Hypnosis, you will see them as allies and not as a burden.

The Downsides of Hypnotherapy for Weight Loss

Like other weight-loss treatments, hypnotherapy also has its disadvantages, albeit these are minor and tolerable ones.

Using Hypnosis to combat obesity is not invasive and usually works well with other treatments for losing weight. You also don't need to take any pills or supplements for the medicine to become effective.

One major downside of hypnotherapy is that it may not work for everyone. According to a Stanford study, 25% of the global population simply can't be placed under Hypnosis, mainly because their brains are wired. This treatment requires the patient to be willing. So, if you feel forced to do it, it may not work for you.

Another downside of using hypnotherapy for weight loss is the price. The cost of a hypnotherapy session per hour may vary depending on where you live, but the range is between $75 and $300 an hour for a session with a professional hypnotherapist.

So, if you get into a session at least once a week or more in a month, it can add up quickly. In addition, most insurance companies will not cover hypnotherapy, so you may have to pay for the sessions from your pocket. But if it is approved as a component of a mental health package, you might be covered, so be sure to check with your insurance provider.

CHAPTER 6:

Lose weight fast and naturally with Hypnosis

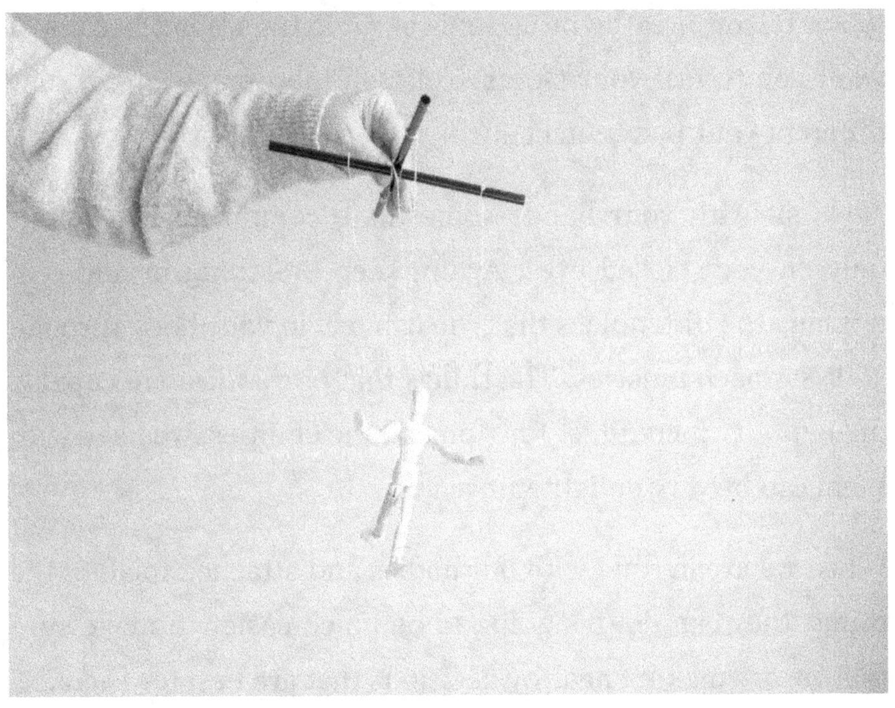

First, start by placing your hand on your stomach. As you do this, feel the body that exists underneath. It's not the one you want right now, but it's the one that you have. As you breathe in, feel your stomach expand.

As you let that air out, feel your stomach flatten. Now, count to five with me as you breathe in. One, two, three, four, five. Count to six as you breathe out. Hold for an extra second because I want you to feel your stomach flatten. Become aware of how different your body can change.

Now, sit with your hands somewhere comfortable, focusing only on your closed eyes. Again, keep breathing in and out, noticing the differences that you can feel in your body through your stomach muscles. The things that our bodies are capable of are pretty incredible. Knowing all the abilities, we have with them can be very enlightening.

When we are in tune with our bodies and attached to all of the things they can do, it's going to be much easier to make sure that we are making healthy decisions that are best for them.

Now, slowly let your mind drift somewhere relaxing. Pick a place in nature. Maybe it's a forest, a beach, or a large grassy field. Wherever it is, I want you to envision this. Now, I'm going to count to ten again, and as I do, your mind is going black. One, two three, four, five, six, seven, eight, nine, ten.

Now, you see nothing but black. As you focus on nothing, a small light emerges, and you see it starting to grow. As it does, you become more relaxed, still feeling the air enter and exit your body. The light keeps going, and before you know it, it is pouring all over your body.

You suddenly realize that you aren't thinking about this place in nature; you are there. As you look around, there is green surrounding you. The blue sky emerges through the leafy green trees, and you can feel the warm sun start to warm your skin.

A cool breeze comes over your body, and you feel the freshness through your hair. You are not afraid of being alone in this place in nature. It is something that you have been waiting for. This is what you deserve.

You start to walk forward, not going anywhere in particular. As you take each step, you begin to see a small building in the distance. You are slowly walking, feeling your body relax. You feel light, fresh, healthy. Something about the way you feel now is different than how you did before.

The building is right in front of you now, and you take it upon yourself to walk in. as you open the door, light pours onto you, and you suddenly feel even more rejuvenated. The building is air-conditioned, and you can tell that it is fresh and new. You aren't sure where you are, but it doesn't matter. No one seems to be there, but you are not afraid to be alone. As you walk in, you see a mirror standing right in front of you.

At first, you are afraid to look into it. There might be a person looking back at you that you do not want to see. Something is telling you that it is time to look into this mirror, however. As you walk up to it, you are shocked to see the person looking back at you. This is a person that you don't recognize at first. They are healthy. They are smiling. Their skin is clear, and their hair is radiant. They are fit, and you can tell that they are working out. The more you look at them, the more you realize that this is you. This is the version that you have been waiting for.

You have had visions in the past of what it might look like if you were to decide to go through with your weight loss journey finally. Now, you are here. You are looking into the mirror and seeing a person that you have been hoping for all along. You are happy and healthy. You are confident, and you are excited.

As you look into the mirror, you suddenly remember all that it took to get there. There were moments where you thought that you couldn't do it. There were times when the only thing that felt right was for you to give up. There were many obstacles in your way, but you finally dared to fight through them and get what you wanted.

As you look at your legs, you see that they are healthy. They carried you for your entire life, helping you get places that you would never have imagined. You can see the outline of your muscles in them, so strong and sleek. As you move up, you see the flat stomach that you have always wanted.

You might still have a few stretch marks, but they are there as a reminder of how much you worked for your health. You fought for yourself for your body. You went through things that others aren't able to do on their own. You see this in your torso. All the food that looked so appetizing that you said "no" to shows in your flat stomach now. Every time you chose something healthy instead of something simply tasty is making itself present in your body.

As you look into the mirror, you see that your chest is strong as well. This healthy chest protects your heart, and you can feel it working well as it sends blood throughout your body. You are feeling energized, correct, fulfilled, and happy. Finally, you see your shoulders and arms. These are so strong and have also helped to carry you so far.

You look at them from your fingers to your neck, toned and supporting the rest of your body. Though you have seen all of the important changes throughout your body, the most important thing is how large your smile is now. Your cheeks are stretched to show the radiance that has always existed inside of you and can finally be present now.

It feels so good to know that you look this good, but what is even better than that is that you are so comfortable with your body.

Throughout your weight loss, you learned how to take care of yourself in a healthy way so that you will be able to keep the weight off for a long time. There were moments when all you wanted was a specific body, but right here, smiling into the mirror, you know now that the most important thing is that you are happy.

It is time now for me to bring you out of the Hypnosis. When I count to ten, you will be back into the present world, ready to start your journey. One, two, three, four, five, six, seven, eight, nine, ten.

Using Hypnosis to Overcome the Mental Barriers

We create habit patterns through repetition, and with time, they become automatic responses to the environment.

Deep in our minds, we have strong ideas that keep us thinking of unhealthy behaviors. Over time, people train the mind to believe that unhealthy behaviors, like emotional eating or overindulging, are necessary to maintain our well-being. And as such, if the mind repeatedly thinks of these behaviors, long-term changes become very difficult.

Emotional eating is just an example of associations that negatively affect our efforts to lose weight.

There are several other associations that people develop, which impact their relationship with food negatively. Some of these associations that hinder weight loss include:

- Food and constant eating help in distracting us from anxiety, anger, and sadness

- Food is a comforting tool; it comforts us when we are feeling sad or stressed

- Overeating sugary or unhealthy foods are associated with good times and celebrations

- Sugary and unhealthy foods are a reward

- Overeating can help one to overcome the fear that you won't manage to lose weight

- Food is a source of entertainment when one is feeling bored

Ultimately, losing weight successfully with Hypnosis requires that we assess these root causes, understand them, and finally reframe them.

This is what Hypnosis can do!

Reframing Your Addiction to Food using Hypnosis

The first step of a hypnosis process is: To identify why you have not achieved your weight loss goals. How does this happen? To understand your shortfalls, a hypnotherapist will typically ask you questions about your eating behaviors and your weight loss journey. This information gathering process will help you identify what you might need to change to attain your goal.

After understanding your eating habits, a hypnotherapist will guide you through an induction process, which entails the relaxation of the mind and body. You will enter a hypnotic state. While in the state, your mind will become highly suggestible; you will have shed off your conscious, critical mind, allowing the hypnotherapist to speak directly to your unconscious mind.

In Hypnosis, you will be provided with positive affirmations and suggestions, and you may be asked to visualize changes. There are several positive suggestions for rapid weight loss, including:

Identify the possible unconscious eating habits—With Hypnosis, you will identify the negative unconscious eating patterns that you have developed over time. When you are hypnotized, you can become more aware of what makes you consume unhealthy food and develop strategies to change the habit.

Reframing your inner voice— with Hypnosis, you will be able to "speak" with the inner voice that misleads you to eat unhealthy food. A hypnotherapist can help you "communicate" with your inner voice. Still, he/she can also turn your inner voice into a support system that guides you to consider positive and rational suggestions.

Developing healthy coping tactics—with Hypnosis, you will develop healthy ways to cope with stress. During Hypnosis, you will become aware that snacking is not the only way to deal with anxiety and stress. You will, therefore, consider other coping strategies.

Improve your food choices— you might be addicted to junk food, but you will develop a low for healthier foods with Hypnosis.

Encouraging healthy eating— With Hypnosis, you will develop the habit of choosing healthier eating habits such as reducing your food portion sizes or rehearsing certain eating choices like taking the remaining food home when you are eating in a restaurant.

Visualizing success— a hypnotic program will encourage you to visualize how you can achieve weight loss goals. Once you visualize how it feels to lose weight, you will have higher chances of practicing the weight-loss tactics.

Improve your confidence— with Hypnosis, and you will develop positive suggestions that boost your self-confidence. With confidence, you will be able to achieve your weight loss goals.

Identifying the unconscious indicators— with hypnotic therapy, you will identify the signals you receive from your body. This can help you understand when you are full and identify the difference between feeling hungry and being thirsty.

When doing Hypnosis, these suggestions can help you to overcome your cravings and poor eating habits. Not all of them apply to every person. However, the goal is to develop a hypnosis plan, which includes the only relevant suggestions.

How Hypnosis helps you Achieve Rapid Weight Loss

During Hypnosis, your mind becomes open to any suggestions. Studies have shown that your brain is likely to experience interesting changes when in the hypnotic state, allowing learning about the information you are receiving without having to think critically or consciously.

In this state, you are always detached from your conscious mind. Thus, you don't interrupt your thoughts with a question about what you are hearing. And this is how Hypnosis helps break down barriers that prevent you from shedding off weight.

In hypnotherapy, repetition is the key to success. This explains why many hypnotherapists provide you with self-hypnosis recordings, which you own to listen to repeatedly.

The brain's barriers are always very strong, and only through repeated Hypnosis can you untangle yourself from the convictions.

Hypnosis teaches the mind how to think differently about eating and food. The suggestions we discussed above can help you achieve the following:

Control Food Cravings

Weight loss hypnotic techniques can help you to detach yourself from cravings and isolate yourself from unhealthy foods. For instance, during Hypnosis, you might be asked to visualize how you will send away the cravings. Suggestions can help in reframing cravings and teach you how to manage them efficiently.

Success

Expectations of an individual dictate his/her reality. With the expectation of success, we are apt to take the steps necessary to attain success.

Hypnosis can plant this seed of success in your mind, thus, giving you the unconscious power to keep yourself on course.

<u>Positivity</u>

Nobody likes negativity, and our brains are no different. Negative thoughts can spoil your ability and dedication to lose weight.

Through Hypnosis, you will become aware of the foods that you "can't eat." These foods do not help your body or health in any way. Thus, hypnotherapy will make you understand that you are not punishing yourself by abstaining from these foods, but you improve your overall being.

<u>Preparing for Relapse</u>

Our minds have been trained to think that relapsing from a journey or goal is a sinful act, as it is a reason to give up. However, Hypnosis gives us the chance of relapsing differently. The relapse becomes an opportunity to examine what went wrong, learn from it, and then prepare for future temptation.

<u>Modifying Behaviors</u>

We can only achieve big goals by taking small steps at a time. Hypnosis empowers us to take the step for these small changes, which eventually result in bigger goals.

For instance, when you always reward yourself with high-calorie content and sugary foods, you will, over time, choose a healthier reward through Hypnosis.

<u>Visualizing Success</u>

Hypnosis is considered a powerful motivator. You might be able to visualize your future-self, telling others how easy it is to lose weight.

Getting Started with Weight Loss Hypnosis

Do you want to start your weight loss journey today? To begin with, you have several different options. One of the options is to visit a certified hypnotherapist who will offer you face-to-face hypnosis sessions. Alternatively, you may schedule a session with a hypnotherapist via a virtual conference. Also, you may consider recorded Hypnosis for self-training. The three common hypnosis options include:

<u>One-on-one hypnosis session</u>

This session helps you to identify the unconscious mental barriers that may hinder you from reaching your goal. Once you acknowledge your obstacles, you will be able to develop effective strategies to overcome them. Below are the things that happen during one-on-one Hypnosis for weight loss: The hypnotherapist will guide you into reaching a state of Hypnosis or deep relaxation. Once you feel fully relaxed, the therapist will be able to access your unconscious mind, including your survival mechanisms and innate instincts.

The hypnotherapist will then use soothing, worded scripts to explore your reasons for overeating and suggest new thinking strategies through visualization. The process enables you to control any of the therapist's suggestions that you are no happy.

Guided hypnosis sessions

This hypnosis technique entails hypnosis sessions that give you the advantage of mobility. You will start the sessions whenever you are ready and always use them when you are on vacation or at home. The recorded sessions can take you through weight loss, including suggestions that are valuable to you.

Self-conducted hypnosis sessions—An advantage of this option is that it is free of charge. The main disadvantage of this approach is that it can be confusing because you may not be aware of what you are doing in the process; thus, you may not meet your weight loss goals.

CHAPTER 7:

Weight loss meditation

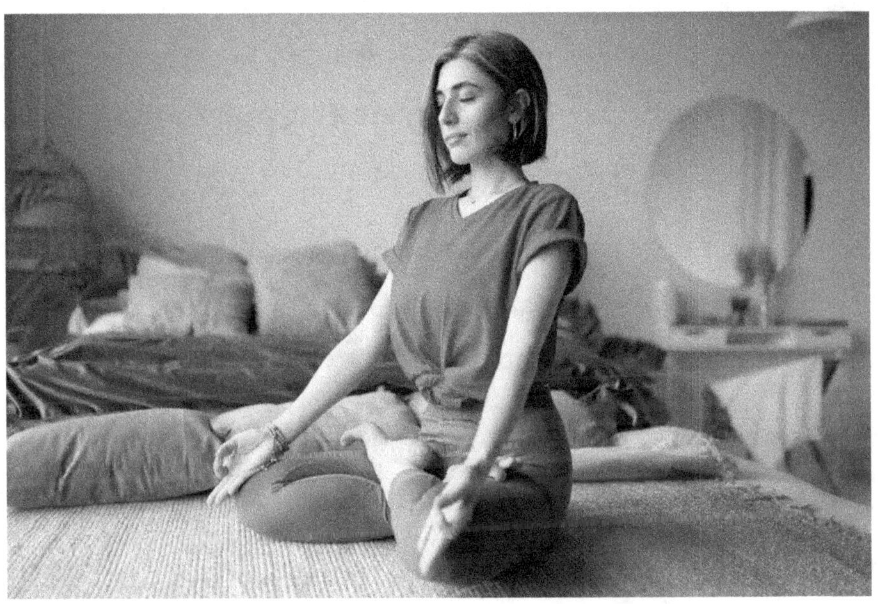

Daily Weight Loss Meditation

Meditation is in fashion. As soon as you tell someone that you have a problem, it is a rare occasion when they do not recommend you practice it. It does not matter if the problem is mental or physical.

Sometimes, people's insistence leads us to reject a plan idea. However, would it not be more interesting to ask why so many people agree to advise you the same thing?

Interest in Eastern cultures brought the influence of ideas to the forefront. And they are our existence's nucleus. Nutrition and physical exercise promote our body's optimal working.

Yet, it is also true that when our emotions aren't controlled, the brain secretes substances that affect our bodies and minds.

Therefore, physical sufferings or thoughts that make life difficult for us can appear. In this way, meditation helps to keep us safe.

Meditation lowered inflammation levels

Beyond what happened in mind, they find an inflammation measure lower than before the investigation. It indicates that perception benefits go beyond what would appear.

The group manager warns that the exact extent of its benefits cannot yet be defined. Nevertheless, the observation is adequate to multiply scientists' efforts in this regard.

It is no longer about Buddhist experiences or self-help customers who can't control.

We have evidence. However, intentional meditation enhances our quality of life. Furthermore, its effects last four months mean that it is a long-term practice that benefits us.

Given the number of harmful elements to which we are exposed, it seems reasonable to bet on this option without being able to do anything.

All this shows us how the first step to improving our health is to listen to our bodies.

It is improbable that the effects you notice when introducing a new habit constitute a mere imagination. Therefore, from here, we want to thank the efforts of many people who have defended an alternative lifestyle—another class of medicine.

Even when they have been treated as "enlightened" and a little sane, their constancy and the defense of their values have been translated into a scientific study that has proved them right and from which we will all benefit.

Practicing anti-stress meditation at home

We know that sometimes it costs. How to combine our daily obligations with that moment of anti-stress meditation? We get up with things to do and arrive at bed with a mind full of those tasks and commitments that must be fulfilled for the following day.

Be careful if the preceding paragraph is an example of what you always live in your day today. You must know how to organize times and set limits, control all those pressures that do not allow you to get rest. Ideally, you learn to balance your life. Where you are always the priority of taking care of your health and emotions, stress can hurt you a lot, and you should see it as an enemy to dominate and do small to handle it properly. We explain how to practice anti-stress meditation.

Emotional agenda

Do you keep a plan in your day to day of the things you should do? Of your obligations, appointments, meetings, appointments with teachers of children, or your visit to the doctor?

Do the same with your emotions, with your personal needs. Spend at least one hour or two hours for yourself each day. To do what you like, to be alone, and to practice anti-stress meditation. Your emotions have priority; make a hole in your day today. You deserve it, and you need it.

A moment of tranquility

It doesn't matter where it is. In your room, in the kitchen or a park.

You must be calm and surrounded by an environment that is pleasant, peaceful, and comforting. If you want, put on the music that you like, but you must be alone.

Regulate your breathing

Let's now take care of our breathing. Once you are comfortable, start to take a deep breath through your nose.

Allow your chest to swell, then let this air out little by little through your mouth.

If you repeat it six or seven times, you will begin to notice a pleasant tingling through your body, and you feel better and calmer.

Focus thoughts

What will we do after? Visualize those pressures that concern you most. Are you pressured at work? Do you have problems with your partner?

Visualize those images and keep breathing. The tension should soften, the nerves should lose their intensity, and the fear will ease. You will feel better little by little.

Positive images

Once you have focused on those images, what more pressure they cause on your being? Let's now visualize pleasant things and aspects that you would like to be living, which would make you happy.

They must be simple things: a walk on the beach; you are touching the bark of a tree, you walk through a quiet city where the sun illuminates your face and where the rumor of nearby coffee shops envelops you with a pleasant smell of coffee. Easy things make you happy. Visualize it and keep breathing deeply.

The silence

Now we close our eyes. At least for two minutes. Try not to think about anything; just let the silence envelop you. You are at peace, and you are well; there is no pressure. There are only you and a peaceful world where there are no pressures and threats, and everything is warm and pleasant.

Open your eyes in a renewed way

It is time to open your eyes and breathe normally again. Look around without moving, without getting up. Don't do it, or you'll run the risk of getting dizzy. Allow about five minutes to pass before you walk again. Indeed you feel much better, lighter, and without any pressure on your body.

New perspectives

Now that you feel more relaxed try to think about what you can do to find yourself better day by day.

Being a little happier sometimes requires that we have to make small changes. And the good thing about anti-stress meditation is that it is slowly changing us inside.

It requires us to make small changes to find the balance so that the body and the mind feel in tune again, and the pressures, the anxieties go out of our body like the smoke that escapes through a window.

Simple Meditation Exercises

Stress accumulates like oil. Paradoxically, as one increases, the other declines. Therefore, stress and energy can fuel a wide variety of sources.

For example, stress may feed on problems in various places or simply a life pattern marked by a lack of breaks. We will present simple meditation exercises to help relieve this stress.

Indeed, meditation encourages self-awareness. It is an ancient Indian peculiar millennial technique, popular in Buddhist and Hindu beliefs. It's become common in the West in recent years.

Focus your attention on breathing

The first of the simple meditation exercises is also one of the easiest to incorporate into our routine. We will do it more easily if we can adopt a relaxed position with semi-open eyes.

It is also good to focus on our breathing without trying to vary the parameters. It's about perceiving the air coming in and going out. At this moment, it is common to be distracted by different thoughts. Our mission will be to ignore them until they lose their strength.

Countdown

This technique is straightforward and is of great use when it comes to meditating. With your eyes closed, count back from high numbers such as 50 or 100 until you reach zero. The goal of this practice is to focus our attention on a single thought/activity. In this way, we will be able to eliminate the sensations produced by the rest of the stimulations.

Scan our own body

This is the most interesting one of many and simple meditation exercises. We only need to reassess the different parts of our body. For this, it is recommended to place ourselves in a place of weak stimulation. Then we will focus our attention on all parts of our body, starting from the head to finish with the feet.

We can contract and release the different muscle groups to become aware of their presence and their movement. It is a rather attractive way to observe ourselves and perceive in detail the sensations of our body.

Observe dynamically

This exercise is focused on studying our climate. Let's start with a comfortable position; the best is sitting with your eyes closed. We'll then open them to approach them for a moment. Before that, we'll have to focus on what's learned.

We'll be able to think about the various sensations that we're generating the stimulations that came to us. We may list them; think of each object's shapes and colors, or name. Furthermore, it might be an excellent way to experience our home differently if we know this at home.

Meditating in motion

Another basic meditation exercise we can put into action is based on our body's feedback of fun stimuli as it moves. For this, interaction with nature is recommended.

For example, we can take a few steps on the beach or in the woods and enjoy the warmth of the sun on our faces, the wind caresses, or the touch of plants and water on our hands. It can also be another way to make a personal observation, thinking about our body's movements as we walk.

<u>Meditate with fire</u>

Finally, we can use fire as a symbolic purification item to focus our meditation. We may concentrate on a campfire in nature or something simpler: a candle's flame. It will allow us to experience the heat sensations associated with fire and the shadows reflecting on the surrounding objects.

On the other side, we can list and burn negative items in our everyday lives. This positive gesture that can be performed symbolically or factually helps us free ourselves from our worries of something we have no influence over.

CHAPTER 8:

Strategies for weight loss

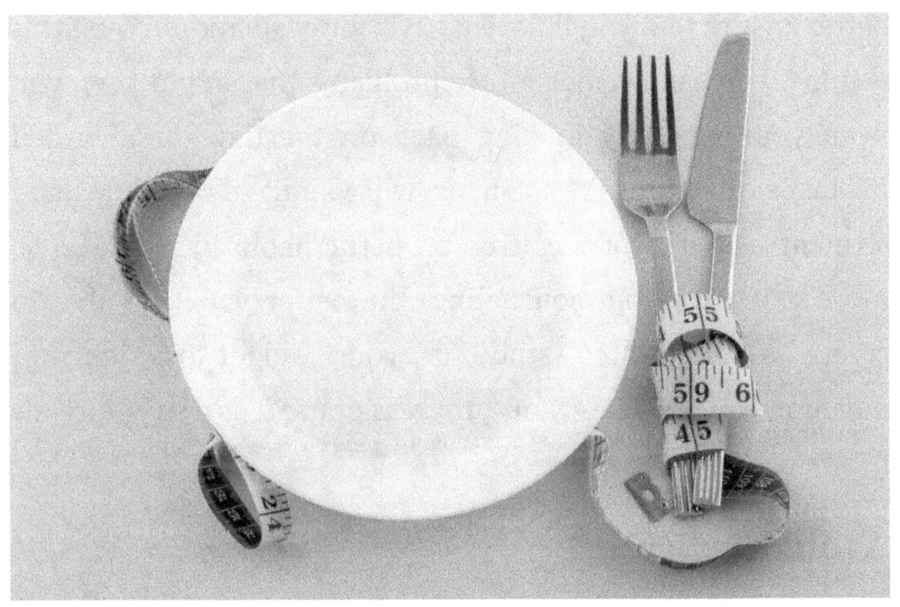

Keep a Journal

Keeping a journey is a healthy habit for many people, no matter their goals, but it's essential for someone that wants to lose weight. By writing down your different portion measurements and exercise habits, you can better ensure that you'll have a basis for evaluation. When this is done, you can predict future problems that might keep you from your goals by looking back on the days of recorded mistakes or slipups. You can see what kinds of schedules and structures aren't working to create better habits in the end. The more extensive your journaling, the better you'll be able to create your research study of your weight-loss journey, meaning you can share your progress or use it as a structure for future diets.

Avoid the Scale

The biggest issue with weight-loss strugglers comes when they see the number on the scale. Someone that wants to lose ten pounds might get discouraged if they find they only lost nine. Sometimes, people might even have to gain weight before they end up losing a pound. By avoiding the scale altogether, certain failures and disappointments can be avoided as well.

Find a different way to track your progress. You can have monthly weigh-ins, but it shouldn't be something that should be checked once a day.

Our weight fluctuates so much throughout our journey that it isn't worth stressing daily. Any checking that happens more than once a day is also likely a bad habit; you're using it to distract yourself from a bigger issue.

The Calorie Myth

When many people diet, they focus too much on calories. They'll see that a specific snack pack only has a hundred calories, which means that it's good for you, right? Wrong. When we focus too much on how many calories are in something, we're failing to look at all the other factors that make up that product. Something with zero calories might include harmful chemicals or hidden substances that are bad for us. Something with a ton of calories might be avoided even though it has many vitamins and necessary fiber.

Calories should still be considered, as the more calories you take in, the more you have to burn through exercise. They always shouldn't be a basis for what foods you decide to eat. If you focus too much on calories, you'll end up losing sight of other important issues.

Remember that weight loss isn't about numbers. What's on the scale or the nutrition package is essential in making specific measurements, but they shouldn't be the definitive goals you're creating on your weight-loss journey.

Affirmations

Practicing affirmations is a vital mindset strategy in weight loss. An affirmation is a type of positive reinforcement that helps in combating negative thoughts. Instead of telling yourself you're "no good" because you didn't follow through with a small goal, you should give yourself an affirmation such as "I am capable of continuing" to remind yourself of how powerful you are. Below is a list of positive affirmations you should use to combat negative thoughts and improve overall encouragement:

- I can do this. I am capable of losing weight, and I can reach my goals.

- I am exercising every day and eating healthy as often as possible. I am doing what I should be doing to achieve my goals.

- If I can start my journey, I can finish it.

- I do not need processed foods to feel happy. I can feel the same joy from cooking a healthy meal.

- I have exercised before and can do it again. It is hard to start, but I know that I have what it takes to finish my exercise routine once I do.

- I am healing myself. I have been through challenging times and deserve to feel happy.

- I am loved and am full of love.

- I am losing weight to be healthy.

- I am beautiful no matter what size. Skipping one day at the gym does not mean that I am not beautiful.

- I am eating healthy food full of nourishment. I can feel the positive change in my body, and I know that I only have more to look forward to.

You control the crucial elements that make self-hypnosis work for you. These elements, which might be motivation, belief, and expectation, are the equal components that give you joy or fulfillment for any aim you choose. Let us look at each element and how you may use it to carry out your hypnosis.

Motivation

Motivation is the electricity for your choice of what you want. Wanting is a feeling that you may control. You have managed your preference or looking through limiting it or denying it in most of your lifestyles. You may be superb at handling your goals and wanting in some regions and susceptible or unpracticed in others.

Since that is a "diet" book, you could have already organized yourself to listen that this "diet" will be just like the others that have informed you what you must deny yourself or limit. I.e., the alternative diets have instructed you what no longer to need, and the emphasis may also have been about "no longer trying" a few foods that you have grown to love. Welcome to a fresh way of treating yourself; we can inspire you to get even higher at "looking." We did not cover denial in this guide.

Your motivation is a crucial factor, and one of the fundamental substances. We want you to focus your strength of looking not closer to food, however closer to the incentive that genuinely tells your mind-body what you want it to create: best weight. We inspire you to get in reality desirable at wanting your perfect weight. Here is an example. Let's say you are in a swimming pool, and abruptly you breathe in a mouthful of water.

Time Is on Your Side

You do now not need to worry about how long any patterns or packages have been running on your unconscious or thoughts-frame. They can exchange the instant you discover what needs correction or realignment, as properly as while you make the deliberate choice to alternate them. We would like you to know how your thoughts-frame is familiar with time. You are aware of the linear and mechanical dimension of time in days, hours, minutes, and seconds—what we call "clock time."

That is the way your conscious mind understands the dimension of time. Your unconscious, your mind-frame, handiest understands "now time," where one minute can appear like ten, or ten minutes can seem like one, or the entire thing is happening in the "now." In your sleep, you could revel in a dream occurring inside the region you lived as a child, but with people who went to your high school, human beings you may see at tomorrow's scheduled meeting, and the person who took your order for lunch that day.

All this could arise at the identical time to your dream because your unconscious perceives all time as "now." During your trance work, you may listen to Dr. G. point out that your unconscious can use the hypnotic pointers along with pics and thoughts of destiny as if they have already occurred. Since all time is "now time" to your subconscious, you can adjust, replace, or create the thoughts and programs that you want to "run" within you right "now."

Changed Forever

Roger Bannister, a British athlete, is an excellent example of a person selected to trust himself. Until 1954, when he broke the document time for going for walks the mile in less than four minutes, the arena believed that it's not possible. Yet within three hundred and sixty-five days of his achievement, thirty-seven other runners around the sector additionally ran the mile in less than four minutes.

When your ideas about something alternate, they do now not revert to old ideals that no longer maintain genuinely. As you make adjustments, adjustments, and realignments for your dreams, they're for all time changed. New beliefs are contagious and unfold rapidly.

Check-in with yourself. Tell yourself that your past enjoyment with a weight-reduction plan and weight loss isn't always a predictor of your achievement. Expect your success by using your motivation, beliefs, and expectations. You will see what you accept as real.

Is It All in Your Mind?

Now you'll be thinking maybe the ideas you are studying about ideals and self-hypnosis are "all on your mind." That is a truthful question. It changed into the normal notion that hypnosis became a psychological revel that most effectively involved the mind.

However, studies show that it involves each of the body and mind. A look at the report inside the American Journal of Psychiatry in 2000 used PET brain scans to look at the regions of the mind activated by shade and gray sunglasses.

They found that after the proven result of hypnotized topics, the gray color had changed into the shade, the elements of the mind that method color got activated, and the gray-color processing areas were not.

Research in Neuro-Image in 2004 used useful MRI mind scanning to look at the parts of the mind activated by using ache. Subjects have been given hypnotic pointers to revel in pain. The researchers located that hypnotically precipitated ache and physically produced ache triggered the same components of the brain.

What these studies tell us is, "Yes, it's far in your mind ... and your body." Your body responds to ideas, thoughts, expectations, and hypnotic hints as real, totally, and physically.

For the foremost part, once we are talking about losing weight and ensuring that we will get our health within the right order that we might like, we are getting to focus on exercise and, therefore, the diet. Both of those are important. One goes to make sure that we are ready to reduce and keep our hearts as healthy as possible within the process and is understood to repel tons of the various diseases out there. But the opposite one will help to scale back weight and make sure the body is getting the nutrients it needs.

Slow Down and Chew

We have to start out slowing down when it's time to eat our meals. We'd like to offer the brain a while to process what you're eating and understand once you have had enough to eat. Once you chew the food all the way through, it's getting to force you to hamper in your eating, and it's getting to be associated back with a decreased amount of food that you simply absorb. It can cause you to feel full faster, and you'll combat smaller portion sizes.

How fast you're ready to finish your meals also can have an enormous effect on your current weight. One review done on 23 observational studies found that the people who ate their meals tons faster were more likely to realize weight than the slower eaters. And fast eaters in these studies were also those who are more likely to be obese.

This is a simple thing to repair. You'll set a timer and not allow yourself to eat faster than that at any time. You'll also make it's found out so that you count what percentage times that you chew each bite, then take a drink of water in between. This is often getting to be a simple thanks for assisting you in hampering and can make it easier to eat less at the meal.

Go With Smaller Plates

You will find that the standard food plate may be a lot bigger than it won't be. This is often a trend that's getting to contribute to weight gain because employing a smaller plate can help you eat less as your portions are getting to look tons larger than they are. This is often an honest thanks to making sure that you're getting to trick your mind about what proportion it eats.

On the opposite hand, once you work with a plate that's tons bigger, it's getting to make a serving, a bigger one, look smaller.

You'll be more likely to feature on more food and eat quite you ought to. This suggests that you simply can use this to your advantage. If you're getting to eat tons of healthy foods, accompany the larger plate, so you're taking on bigger portions of it and obtain more of those great things. But if you're getting to eat foods that aren't as healthy, then plow ahead and accompany the smaller plates.

Add within the Protein

Protein goes to possess some powerful effects on appetite. It's ready to help us increase our feelings of fullness, scale back your hunger, and make it easier to eat fewer calories. This might be because protein affects several hormones that play a hunger and fullness task, including the ghrelin hormone.

There is one study that found once we increase our protein intake from 15 percent to 30 percent of our calories, it made it easier for participants to require 441 fewer calories per day then lose 11 pounds over 12 weeks on average, and this was all without intentionally restricting any of the opposite foods that the participants were eating. A good thanks to using this is often together with your meals. If you're eating a breakfast that's filled with grains, for instance, then switching to a meal that's higher in protein could also be an honest place to start. One study found that obese and overweight women who had eggs as a part of their breakfast were ready to eat fewer calories at lunch than those at breakfast based more on grains.

Eat the Fiber

Eating foods rich in fiber is different for us to form sure that we increase our satiety, which helps us feel fuller for an extended period of your time. Studies also show us that one sort of fiber, which is understood as viscous fiber, goes to help when it involves weight loss. This one is so good because it's ready to increase the quantity of fullness that we've, and it's ready to reduce the foods that we intake.

Drink Water Often

We even have to form sure that we are drinking enough water daily because this may help us refill our stomachs so that we eat less and reduce within the process. This is often getting to happen even more once we confirm to drink before a meal. One study in adults found that drinking about 17 ounces of water about half an hour before a meal would help to scale back the quantity of hunger that was felt and help reduce what percentage calories the individual was getting to absorb.

During this study, those who took the time to drink more water before their meals were ready to lose 44 percent more weight over three months than those who didn't have the water before their meals. If you're prepared to replace a number of the regular drinks that you wish to have, which are loaded with calories, like juice or soda, with water, the load loss that you only are experiencing may be going to be even higher.

Keep the Portions Small

In addition to those bigger plates that we were talking about before, you'll find that portion sizes have seen a rise over the past few decades, especially once we leave to eat. These larger portions encourage people to eat more and maybe linked back to an increase in weight and obesity overall.

One study in adults found that when the appetizer with the dinner was doubled, it had been ready to increase the number of calories taken in by 30 percent. You'll find that serving yourself just a touch bit less might be enough to assist you to eat fewer calories, and if it impossible that you simply would even notice the difference.

Don't Eat Neat the TV

Paying more attention to what you're eating could assist you to require fewer calories overall. Those that eat while they're on the pc or watching a show could easily lose track of the quantity they're eating. This is often getting to cause them to overeat also. One review of 24 studies found that those that were distracted once they were eating their meals would consume about 10 percent more during that sitting than those that paid attention.

Besides, being absent-minded when it came to the meal would significantly influence what proportion you took in later within the day. Those that were more distracted during a meal would eat 25 percent more calories at later meals than those that paid more attention. If you're within the habit of consuming meals while watching TV or using some quiet device, then it's likely you're eating more without noticing. These are calories that will add up and may have an enormous impact on your weight over time.

Try to Avoid Stress and Sleep More

Now, if you're a parent, you almost certainly read the thing above and began laughing. Sleeping well and avoiding all of the strain can seem almost impossible once you are a parent, and you've got a bunch of things to stay track of for your children. And if your children aren't sleeping through the night yet, getting that sleep that you simply need could seem almost impossible also. This is often also why tons of oldsters are getting to gain weight when taking care of their children, and it's a real example of why we'd like to pay a touch more attention to our sleeping styles to make sure that we get enough.

Cut Out the Sugary Drinks

Added sugar goes to be one of the worst ingredients that we are ready to increase our diets today. Numerous studies mention how sugary beverages, like soda, are increasing the danger that we've of the many different diseases. It's very easy to consume more calories from these drinks because the calories from a liquid aren't getting to affect our levels of fullness within the same way that a solid food can

These are just a couple of the items that we are ready to neutralize to scale back the quantity that we are eating daily. Once we are ready to make sure that we are just taking within the great things and reducing the amount of the bad stuff that we are consuming, we are getting to see some big changes in our overall health in no time in the least.

These are all simple tasks that you are ready to try and aren't meant to be difficult or too hard to follow. But once we make a couple of small changes, maybe just trying out one or two of those at a time and slowly build-up, we'll find that it's easier than ever to travel through and lose the load that we would like, regardless of what quite a diet plan we are on within the first place.

CHAPTER 9:

Self-hypnosis for extreme weight loss

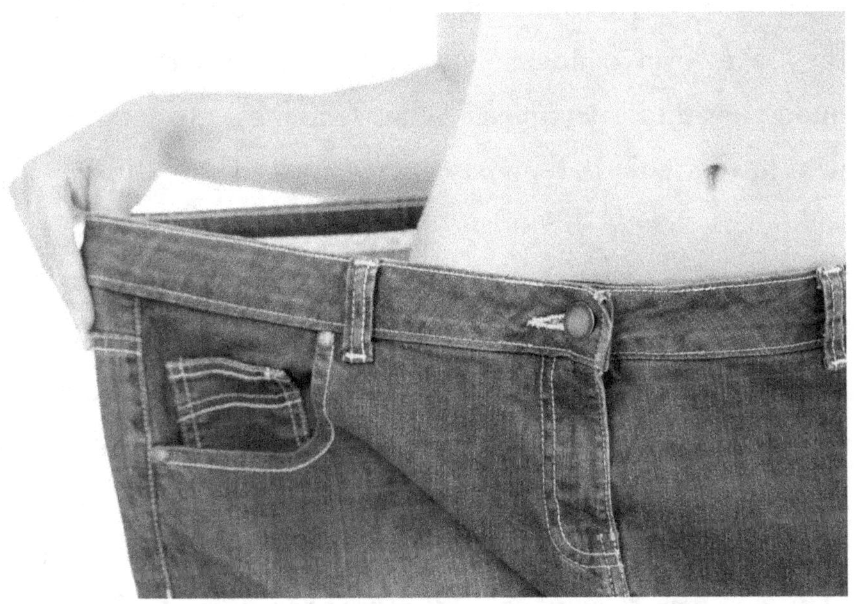

One might ask, "How does hypnosis work?" the solution to the present question isn't definite. The mind has been an enormous puzzle among scientists, and a particular psychological state called Hypnosis may also be a puzzle. The only things that can be said about Hypnosis are the very things that happen in the hypnotic state. These are the behavioral changes and brain activities that a subject undergoes under Hypnosis. What remains a mystery for those who have studied Hypnosis 200 years ago can still be safely said. The term "hypnosis" can be best described as an interaction between two people. If one of the people is trying to influence other people's perceptions, feelings, thinking, and behavior, then the former is called "hypnotist" and the latter the "subject." In this interaction, the hypnotist will ask the subject to concentrate on ideas and images that may evoke the intended responses. The verbal communications that the hypnotist uses to achieve these responses are named "hypnotic suggestions." If a person practiced the hypnotic procedures independently without a hypnotist's help, that activity is called "self-hypnosis."

How Self-Hypnosis Works

Performing self-spellbinding is as basic as having the option to move into a perspective you are in when you are dreaming and resting. The conscious mind in this state is relaxed, and your thoughts can flow freely to and from the subconscious.

Doing this can assist us with a wide range of things. Not exclusively will it assist us with accelerating our weight reduction. However, it can help with sorrow, mending wounds, expanding confidence, assembling a superior body, recuperating inner wounds, relieving disorders, and lots more.

The process is very easy to perform; to begin, locate a decent, calm spot to plunk down, don't rest since you could nod off, and we don't need that to occur. Self-spellbinding for weight reduction can be unwinding and can make us nod off on the off chance that we are not cautious. We will likely have the option to speak with our inner mind. If we are dozing, at that point, this won't occur.

So, when you are plunking down in a suitable position, you can be perched on a seat if this feels the most suitable or on the floor; the best position is one where you are leaning against a divider with your legs loosened up before you.

This position permits you to keep your back straight and feel the vitality stream from your toes to your head; sitting on a seat will also help. In any case, the progression of vitality will be, to some degree, limited due to the bowed knees.

After you are in your agreeable position, loosen up your appendages' entirety and take three full breaths. This causes us to unwind and prepare for our excursion into ourselves.

Next, start by taking a gander at your toes and envision they are loose. Imagine you can see vitality moving upwards from your toes toward your legs.

How to Change Your Thoughts

In the relaxed, attentive state of self-hypnosis, you can be more aware of what are usually "automatic" thoughts. One approach is to use one session to notice and remember the automatic ideas that come up around a particular issue and then write down the thoughts and counter-thoughts you would like to replace them with.

For example, if one of your automatic thoughts was "I never succeed at anything," a counter-thought might be, "I succeed at things often. When I do, I pay attention to them and congratulate myself."

Then, in a second session, you can practice saying the pair of thoughts and gradually shifting the weight of credibility and commitment to the counter-thought.

How to Change Your Feelings

Changing emotions is very feasible with self-hypnosis. A straightforward technique is to connect with the feeling, give it a name (such as "anxiety"), and then notice how it feels in your body.

Imagine what color it would be if it had a color, what texture it would have if it had a texture, what sound it might make. Then imagine that color, texture, or sound changing to one that is more pleasant. Another emotional technique is to imagine your negative feeling on the one hand and a positive feeling you want to replace it with on the other hand. Focus attention on them alternately, gradually bring them together and allow the positive attitude to be dominant as you close your hands together.

How to Change Your Behavior

In self-hypnosis, you can also visualize your future behavior as different from what you currently do in a particular set of circumstances. This mental pre-rehearsal or "future pacing" helps to prepare your mind to behave in that way in real life.

You can also motivate yourself by picturing the positive consequences of changing and comparing them with the negative effects of staying the same.

How to Achieve Your Dreams

If you're clear in your mind about your dreams, you'll have some idea about the thoughts, feelings, and behaviors that belong to someone who's fulfilled those dreams. When you use self-hypnosis to move closer to being that kind of person, your dreams come closer to your grasp.

Emotional Side of Weight Loss and Why It's So Important

Calories in ought to be less than calories out - this is frequently affirmed to be the exact and successful equation of weight reduction. The issue is that the technique doesn't work for some individuals. A solitary explanation exists for that reality - this recipe doesn't factor in the passionate parts of getting in shape.

For some individuals, shedding pounds is a major battle. It incorporates longings, passionate eating, and addictions to specific nourishments. These parts make it inconceivably hard to adequately present change and keep up a person's degree of joy and fulfillment.

Is it true that you are battling with your weight reduction goals? You aren't the only one! A few elements could add to your disappointment, and disregarding the enthusiastic parts of weight addition and misfortune could likewise cause your issues.

The Most Powerful Emotional Components

Several emotional responses could interfere with losing weight and maintenance efforts. The most important ones include:

Anxiety and nervousness: for a few people, these feelings cause enthusiastic eating. When feeling apprehensive, these people need an outlet and a wellspring of solace. Food is much of the time in this outlet. Food "perks up" these people and empowers them to keep working while at the same time holding the adverse feelings within proper limits. Exercise phobia: a passionate component that is regularly thought little of. Numerous individuals accept that activity is unimaginably unpleasant. Some stress over getting to the rec center because of their current weight. They lack motivation, never enjoyed sports, and believe that the situation isn't going to be much different this time. Body image: how do you perceive yourself? The lack of confidence and love for yourself could prevent you from getting to that ideal weight. You may think that you simply don't deserve change or aren't ok to possess a healthy and fit body. This is why you're probably sabotaging your weight loss efforts.

Previously mentioned are not many of the normal intense subject matters remaining inside the fruitful weight reduction method. For certain individuals, it could be much increasingly convoluted. An awful connection with food, compulsion, and reliance is a significantly increasingly genuine mental issue that makes weight reduction unimaginable.

Then Why Do People Fear Hypnosis?

Something that causes individuals to delay utilizing a trance inducer or to utilize self-mesmerizing is that they imagine that entrancing is risky. Indeed, in all cases, the response to this inquiry is that mesmerizing isn't risky. Part of what people seek once they are looking to use a hypnotist is to seek someone who will make them do something they cannot do or don't want.

Furthermore, this idea that they could have this sort of relationship with someone else likewise frightens them. The trance inducer can't transform you into a reluctant member in anything! The trance inducer can just help you with what you're willing and prepared to achieve.

Working with a hypnotist will help you see, feel, and act fully congruent with what you want to accomplish. There's no danger in seeking the assistance of a hypnotist or using self-hypnosis techniques to help you briefly or future goals.

The Key to Making Self-Hypnosis Work

Self-hypnosis has been employed by an excellent many of us to make real, measurable changes in themselves and their lives. Immense quantities of individuals have used the office of self-spellbinding to dispense with fears, control torment, treat physical and mental manifestations, as well as utilizing it to prevail in their objectives.

Notwithstanding, numerous others have accomplished nothing advantageous from its utilization even though specialists state that everybody is hypnotizable! All in all, the inquiry remains - Why doesn't it generally work?

Many people fail to achieve any measurable results from self-hypnosis because they're not using it correctly!

The initial step you should take when considering utilizing self-entrancing is to comprehend what you might want. Despite the fact that this may sound rudimentary and a bit of deigning, truly think about it. Do you know correctly, directly down to the last detail, what you might want to acknowledge from your self-spellbinding project? Or, do you listen to a generic self-hypnosis session and hope for the best?

For example, taking note of a self-hypnosis recording for more confidence could also be an honest goal, but how does one quantify confidence? Do you want to be confident around people or potential mates? It is sheltered to state that you are attempting to recognize more trust in your movement or work-life? Is it actually that you need to be progressively sure about your capacities, and in this way, it is your confidence that you wish to construct?

For self-hypnosis, like all other self-improvement techniques, to be effective, you want to use it with a goal in mind! Your objective, to be utilized with self-mesmerizing, must be exact.

Take a stab at recording a rundown of things you might want to accomplish and afterward organize them. Take your most fundamental want and switch it into an objective. Might you be able to record it? Kindly do it now!

Weight Loss Self Hypnosis

In a supersized world, individuals have numerous chances to eat and drink WAY excessively, yet what's behind corpulence usually is more than longing for a huge request of fries. In America, a genuine eating regimen industry has developed around obesity.

It powers overweight individuals to follow through on a significant expense in vogue diets, pills, or costly and high-hazard medical procedures. By doing away with starches or fat, taking pills or infusions, sprinkling gems on your food, falling back on careful medication, or drinking naturally occurring diet elixirs, numerous health food nuts briefly lose pounds don't lose the outlook which contributes to weight gain.

The outcome is that after such difficult work and conceivably burning through a huge number of dollars, most calorie counters recover their weight and feel significantly progressively disheartened. Weight loss hypnosis can help you change how you feel and control your bad dieting habits.

Why Self-Hypnosis Is A Great Weight Loss Approach

As a whole, we have harmful convictions that impact how we act and think and our practices. A portion of these particular convictions and examples of reasoning to a great extent decide your weight. These could incorporate your disposition toward food and good dieting.

When you make a decent attempt to lose weight, but you are not losing a lot, debilitation makes it simpler to defend droop the cart. You believe, "I'm not losing in any case, so I'd likewise have that hot fudge dessert." Or, "I didn't practice today, so simply overlook it - the week is destroyed."

Weight misfortune mesmerizing trains you to think like flimsy individuals, settle on food choices like these individuals, and eat meager individuals. Despite some reasoning, normally flimsy individuals aren't that way since they generally eat chicken and serve mixed greens with no dressing.

Instead, they recognize what might feel great in their stomachs BEFORE they eat. At that point, they can eat what they need with some restraint and realize when to quit eating depending on how they feel, and see treats as incidental little extravagances, not a day by day need of shoddy nourishment that they later feel sincere and genuinely lousy about eating.

Weight reduction hypnosis advances safe weight reduction. It keeps your mentality positive, in any event, when weight reduction is delayed now and again. While the weight reduction will consistently change a little from week to week, different aftereffects of Hypnosis, for example, developed confidence, unwinding, inspiration, and a quiet perspective, keep on growing. Entrancing changes the association between food and feelings as it re-makes legitimate views toward eating. Since the program doesn't depend on medications and no eating regimens of any sort, Hypnosis is a sound way to deal with weight reduction that can leave you slimmer, progressively loose. With significant changes way, you approach food and your feelings.

Similarly, as with all Hypnosis, the vast majority of individuals can answer recommendations made once they are in a relaxed state. A legitimate trance specialist will assess whether you're the correct contender for weight reduction spellbinding depending on the quality of your craving to change and your readiness to acknowledge preparing and adhere to directions.

CHAPTER 10:

How to use meditation to beat food cravings

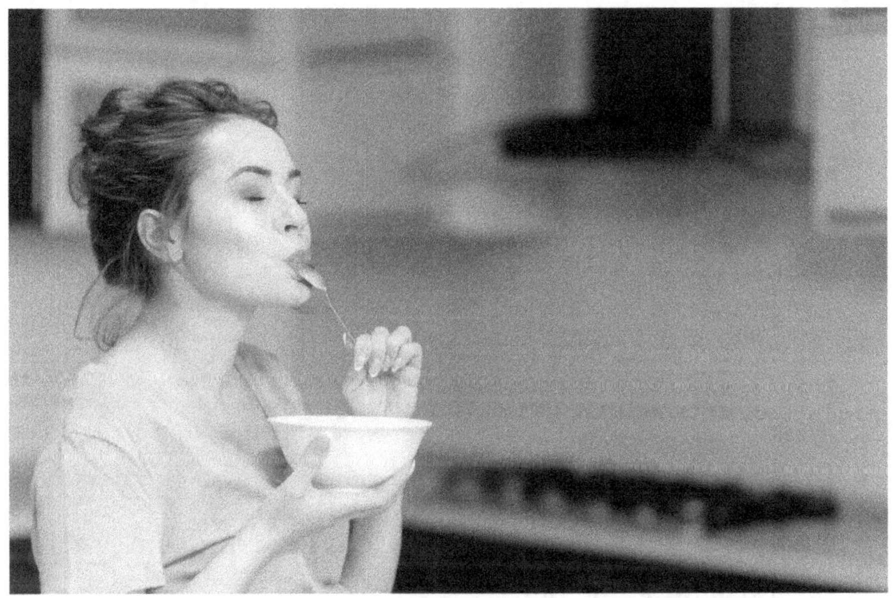

Meditation

Meditation is an activity that helps create a sense of relaxation by linking the body and mind. As a spiritual activity, individuals have been meditating for centuries. Most individuals today use meditation to relieve tension and become more mindful of their emotions.

There are various ways of meditation. A few are focused on the usage of mantras named particular phrases. Others concentrate on the moment of breathing or maintaining consciousness.

Like how the mind and body function, these approaches will help you gain a deeper understanding of yourself.

This enhanced sensitivity allows meditation a valuable technique that might aid in weight reduction and further appreciate your eating patterns.

What's the Link Between Losing Weight and Meditation?

An important method to assist people in losing weight, maybe meditation. What precisely makes meditation in that sense so powerful? It coincides with the unconscious and conscious brain to settle on adjustments we want to add to our actions. These adjustments may involve the regulation of cravings for junk food and the alteration of eating patterns. Having the unconscious mind engaged is crucial since unhealthy, weight-gaining habits such as comfort eating are rooted. Meditation will help you be more mindful about these and overcome them with meditation and substitute them with weight loss practices.

Although meditating provides a more urgent benefit. "The quantities of stress hormones may be decreased explicitly by meditation. Stress hormones like cortisol send our bodies a signal to accumulate energy as fat. When you have a lot of cortisol running into your bloodstream, even though you are making healthier decisions, it would be impossible to lose weight. It sounds difficult, we know; we're all tired, and it seems difficult to undo. But all it takes, a report from Carnegie Mellon University showed, is 25 minutes of mediation three days in a row to relieve tension dramatically.

In reality, volunteers in a 2016 study demonstrated "increased concentration, happiness, calmness, body-mind perception, and brain activation" after only a few short sessions. With everyday practice, self-control may also improve, the study indicates. Researchers discovered that those that enable us to regulate ourselves were the areas of the mind most impacted by meditation. That implies that a few mins of meditation regularly will make it a lot easier to skip that next cookie or skip the ice cream when you feel low.

Knowing the terms regarding weight reduction meditation

Unique strategies and techniques—Meditation, conscientious feeding, and intuitive feeding may help us understand or relearn how to establish a healthier interaction with food and reduce any uncomfortable emotions we could have about nutrition. Losing weight can be a side effect of nurturing this revived friendship, but it is crucial not to develop the primary objective of losing weight. Using so will hinder us such that we cannot feed intuitively or in a deliberate manner.

Instead, reflect on enjoying food, feeding because you need to eat, not because you're exhausted and depressed with work or family problems. You can learn how to respect and value your body and what it can do for you through these lessons.

It will help clarify what the language entails when learning about meditation for losing weight or meditation for nutrition and maintaining a healthier attitude towards food.

Panic or emotional feeding arises when individuals, rather than reacting to their internal signals of hunger, prefer to feed and overeat because of intense emotions or thoughts. Perhaps these thoughts will overshadow our actual sensations of contentment and satiation while we encounter intense emotions, which may contribute to our overeating. Food is used as a calming strategy in these situations, dulling intense feelings temporarily.

However, understanding that this event leads to the perpetuation of a pattern is essential. Experiencing stressful feelings may contribute to overeating, which contributes to remorse or embarrassment, going back to experiencing unpleasant emotions or tension, and not managing or maintaining such situations. Mindful eating is a strategy or process that you may utilize to improve your interaction with food and feeding memories. It requires us to be present and activate our senses, how food tastes, feels, and how it makes our bodies react, most significantly. Mindful eating requires intuitive eating to make us calm down and respond to our inner signals of real desire or signals of pleasure, which will make us limit or even entirely avoid our mental or excessive eating. Even though conscious eating will contribute to weight loss, the objective result or incentive should not lose weight. If our dietary decisions are made based on a certain tangible effect we like, it means that we have already quit actively feeding.

A mind-body, non-diet solution to wellbeing and nutrition is intuitive feeding. To heal our attitude towards food, it opposes the idea of dieting and encourages us to embrace our bodies and respond to our internal bodily signs. Intuitive eating involves conscious eating concepts; however, it also contains a broader generalized concept that extends throughout, pushing the body because it feels nice to walk, often without judgment utilizing diet evidence.

When Exercise and Diet Don't Seem To Be Effective, How Will Meditation Help?

Stress is the leading cause of unnecessary weight gain or the failure to lose weight successfully in certain situations. But, if you've been eating correctly and exercising but are continually anxious, you may not be tackling the core reason for weight gain.

Stress again activates hormones that accumulate excess fat, just what we don't like! This can also fuel a tension cycle: when you're anxious, you can't lose weight, which leaves you frustrated over not reaching your goal. Being caught in a simple process, but you can crack it, and meditation can assist.

It would be best to consider what triggers stress in your life to cope with tension or remove it properly.

Few stressors are easy to spot, but others may be more elusive. I consider utilizing Well Be to grasp better, map, and deal with tension.

The WellBe is a device that acts much like a sensor of movement, but now it is the first of its sort to concentrate on mental health. It also shows you how and what behaviors in your life induce emotional tension and will also support you come up with better coping strategies that will help you lose weight.

How to Meditate

There are lots of ways of meditating.

Most forms of meditation have the following four points in common:

- A quiet place. Can you decide where to meditate — your preferred chair? During a walk? It depends on you.

- A certain relaxed pose, such as lying, sitting, standing, or moving.

- A focus of awareness. You may concentrate on a phrase or expression, your breathing, or anything else.

- A transparent mind. Getting other thoughts when you meditate is natural. Try not to be drawn in those feelings so much. Continue to put your focus back to your voice, word, or something else you're focused on.

- Pick the location you want to try, the time, and the process. To understand the fundamentals, you may even take a lesson.

Instantly, meditation won't help you lose weight.

But it will have lifelong impacts on not just your weight but also your thinking processes with a little practice.

Loss of Sustainable Weight

You can recognize all of these things through mindfulness meditation without judgment.

Meditation is related to several advantages. In terms of weight reduction, mindfulness meditation appears to be the most beneficial. A 2017 study of current research showed that mindfulness meditation was a successful tool for weight reduction and improving eating behaviors.

Meditation for Mindfulness means paying careful attention to:

- Where you are

- Whatever you do,

- The way you feel at the current moment.

- Learn to handle your acts and emotions as they are, nothing more. Take inventory of what:

- You experience and do but strive not to categorize something as fair or poor. Through daily practice, everything gets simpler.

Exercising mindfulness meditation may contribute to long-term effects, too. As per the 2017 study, many who cultivate mindfulness are more likely to hold the weight off relative to other dieters.

Methods of meditation

Conscious Meditation.

It's easy to get caught up in a loop of spinning thoughts — starting to think about a laundry list of activities to do, ruminating about past events, or potentially future situations — and practicing mindfulness may help. Yet what exactly is attention? It can be described as a mental state that requires being fully engaged on "the now" so that, without judgment, you can understand and acknowledge your thoughts, feelings, and sensations.

Mindfulness meditation

Mindfulness meditation is the method of having your thoughts fully present. Knowledge involves being mindful of where we are and what we do and not being too sensitive to what is happening around us.

One can do reflective meditation anywhere. Some people like to sit in a quiet spot, close their eyes, and focus on their respiration. But at every stage of the day, even when driving to work or doing chores, you can choose to be conscious.

You track your thoughts and feelings while practicing mindfulness meditation but let them move without judgment.

Directed Meditation.

Directed meditation, often also referred to as guided imagery or visualization, is a meditation technique in which you create mental images or scenarios that you find calming.

Guided meditation is among the most common methods of meditation employed every day by millions of people. In this post, we'll explore guided meditation and how to do it.

In the purest form, guided meditation is a type of meditation where the individual is guided on every step of his daily practice. Someone directs you right from the first level of sitting in a meditative pose to the final phase of completing the meditation. What occurs is that during meditation, a teacher or mentor provides step-by-step guidance about what to do. It is an ancient method of conveying directions for meditation to pupils. In older times, this technique has been used to teach meditation in a group. Nowadays, thanks to technological development, we no longer need a guru's physical presence to lead us in meditation. We can listen to a master's direct guidance using pre-recorded CDs or DVDs and conduct our meditation practice. In the absence of any meditation master professional CDs / DVDs, you can record guided meditation instructions from a book in your voice and then play them afterward.

Vipassana Meditation.

Vipassana meditation is an ancient form of Indian meditation, which means seeing things as they are. More than 2,500 years ago, it was taught in India. The conscious meditation movement has origins in this practice in the United States.

The purpose of meditation with vipassana is self-transformation through the examination of oneself. This is accomplished to create a deep connection between mind and body by careful attention to the body's sensations. The sustained interconnectedness leads to a happy account, filled with love and compassion.

Vipassana is usually taught during a 10-day course in this tradition. People are expected to follow a set of rules all the time and abstain from all intoxicants, telling lies, cheating, sexual activity, and killing any animals.

Loving Meditation on Compassion (Metta Meditation).

Metta meditation, also called meditation on loving-kindness, is the practice of guiding good wishes towards others.

Those who practice reciting similar words and phrases will elicit warm-hearted sentiments. This is also commonly found in meditation on mindfulness and vipassana.

It's usually done in a pleasant, relaxed position while sitting. After a few deep breathes, you slowly and steadily repeat the following words. "Just let me be happy. May I be fine. Let me be free. May I be calm and at ease". After a period of guiding this loving-kindness to yourself, you may begin to imagine a family member or friend who has supported you and repeat the mantra, this time replacing " I " with" you." As you continue the meditation, you may bring to mind other members of your family, friends, neighbors or people in your life. Practitioners are often encouraged to consider individuals who are having trouble with them.

Meditation Yoga.

The yoga practice has its roots in ancient India. There are various yoga classes and styles, but all include performing a series of postures and guided breathing exercises designed to encourage flexibility and relax the mind.

The poses require balance and attention, and practitioners are encouraged to concentrate less on distractions and remain more at the moment.

Which meditation style you choose to try depends on several factors. When you have a health problem and are new to yoga, tell your doctor what method would be right for you

CHAPTER 11:

What is mindful eating

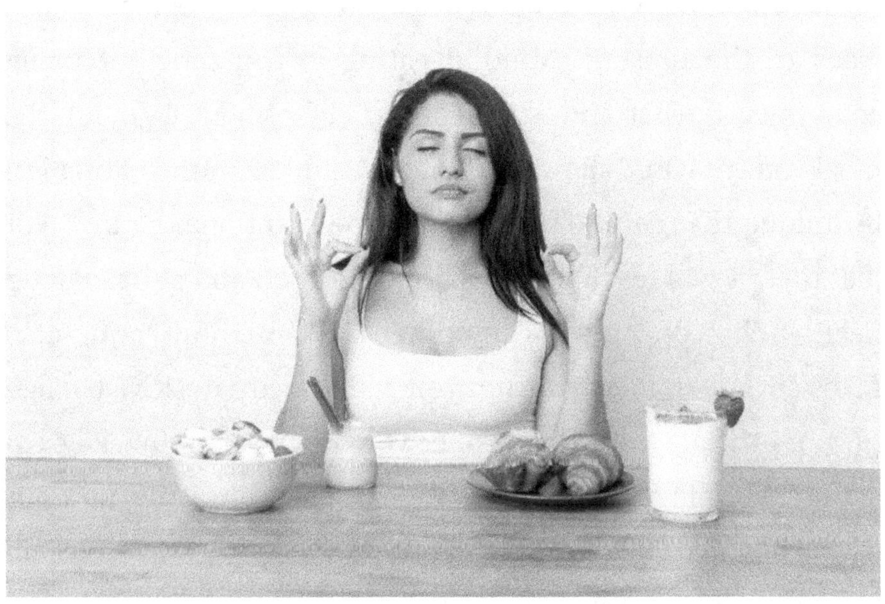

Mindfulness is a simple concept that states that you must be aware of and present in the moment. Often, our thoughts tend to wander, and we might lose track of the present moment. Maybe you are preoccupied with something that happened or are wondering about something that might occur. When you do this, you tend to lose track of the present. Mindful eating is a practice of being conscious of what and when you eat. It is about enjoying the meal you eat while showing some restraint. Mindful eating is a technique that can help you overcome emotional eating. Not just that, it will teach you to enjoy your food and start making healthy choices. As with any other skill, mindful eating also takes a while to inculcate, but you will notice a positive change in your attitude toward food once you do. In this, you will learn about a couple of simple tips you can use to practice mindful eating in your daily life.

Reflection

Before you start eating, take a minute and reflect upon how and what you are feeling. Are you experiencing hunger? Are you feeling stressed? Are you bored or sad? What are your wants, and what do you need? Try to differentiate between these two concepts. Once you are done reflecting for a moment, you can now choose what you want to eat, if you do want to eat and how you want to eat.

Sit Down

It might save some time if you eat while you are working or while traveling to work. Regardless of what it is, you must ensure that you sit down and eat your meal.

Please don't eat on the go, instead set a couple of minutes aside for your mealtime. You will not be able to appreciate the food you are eating if you are trying to multitask. It can also be quite difficult to keep track of all the food you eat when eating on the go.

No Gadgets

If all your attention is focused on the TV, your laptop, or anything else that comes with a screen, it is unlikely that you will be able to concentrate on the meal that you are eating. When your mind is distracted, you tend to indulge in mindless eating. So, limit your distractions or eliminate them if you want to practice mindful eating.

Portion your Food

Don't eat straight out of a container, a bag, or a box. When you do this, it becomes rather difficult to keep track of the portions you eat, and you might overindulge without even being aware of it. Not just that, you will never learn to appreciate the food you are eating if you keep doing this.

Small Plates

We are all visual beings. So, if you see less, your urge to eat will also decrease. It is a good idea to start using small plates when you are eating.

You can always go back for a second helping, but this is a simple way to regulate the quantity of food you keep wolfing down.

Be Grateful

Before you dig into your food, take a moment, and be grateful for all the labor and effort that went into providing the meal you are about to eat.

Acknowledge that you are lucky to have the meal you do, which will help create a positive relationship with food.

Chewing

It is advised that you must chew each bite of food at least thirty times before swallowing it. It might sound tedious but make it a point to chew your food at least ten times before you swallow.

Take this time to appreciate the flavors, textures, and taste of the food you are eating. Apart from this, when you thoroughly chew the food before swallowing, it helps with better digestion and absorption of food.

Clean Plate

You don't have to eat everything that you serve on your plate. I am not suggesting that you must waste food. If you have overfilled your plate, don't overstuff yourself. You must eat only what your body needs and not more than that. So, start with small portions and ask for more helpings. Overstuffing yourself will not do you any good, and it is equivalent to mindless eating.

Prevent Overeating

It is important to have well-balanced meals daily. You shouldn't skip any meals, but it doesn't mean that you should overeat. Eat only when you feel hungry and don't eat otherwise. Here are a couple of simple things you can do to avoid overeating. Learn to eat slowly. It isn't a new concept, but not many of us follow it. We are always in a rush these days. Take a moment and slow down. Take a sip of water after every couple of bites and chew your food thoroughly before you gulp it down. Don't just mindlessly eat and learn to enjoy the food you eat. Concentrate on the different textures, tastes, and flavors of the food you eat. Learn to savor every bite you eat and make it an enjoyable experience. Make your first-bit count and let it satisfy your taste buds. Now is the time to let your inner gourmet chef out! Use a smaller plate while you eat, and you can easily control your portions. Stay away from foods that are rich in calories and wouldn't satiate your hunger. Fill yourself up with foods that can satisfy your appetite and make you feel full for longer. If you have a big bowl of salad, you will feel fuller than you would if you have a small bag of chips. The calorie intake might be the same for both these things, but the hunger you will feel afterward differs.

The idea is to fill yourself up with healthy foods before you think about junk food. While you eat, make sure that you turn off all electronic gadgets. You tend to lose track of the food you eat while you watch TV.

Practicing Mindfulness

Mindfulness meditations help you put some space between yourself and how you react whenever you face any situation. The following practices will guide you to tune into mindful meditation daily:

Set aside some time - All you need is to set aside some time from your busy schedule to engage in meditations. Getting off other activities is the most crucial requirement for effective mindful mediation. Observe your present moment as it is - The goal of mindfulness is to give close consideration to what you are encountering at the immediate moment without judging it. It is not about quieting your mind or attempting to achieve some state of long-lasting calm.

Focus on the sensations, thoughts, and imaginations of your mind at that present moment.

Let your judgments pass - In case you notice any thoughts during your practices, you shouldn't suppress them. Instead, take a mental note of them and let them pass.

Return to the present moment - Once your judgments have passed, focus back your mind to the present, making observations of the current as it is. Mindfulness is about returning your thoughts to the present, sometimes several, during your entire practice.

Your mind tends to carry off easily by the myriads of thoughts crossing it. You must refocus your mind on the present thought.

Don't judge your wandering - You shouldn't be hard on yourself every time your mind wanders off during the practice. It is common for all humans to have thoughts propping up instinctively, and without any warning, you should, therefore, learn how to recognize when your mind wandered off to bring it back and refocus it on the present gently.

Important Mindfulness Techniques

We can practice mindfulness in different ways.

All of the available methods focus on how you can achieve a state of alertness and relaxation to focus your attention on your thoughts and sensations without judging them. The following are some of the meditation techniques:

Basic mindfulness technique

This technique requires you to sit quietly in the same spot and focus on your breathing. You can also focus on saying a single word that you silently say over and over again. You should allow your thoughts to come in and out without judgment, and each time, you return to your focus on the breath.

Body sensations

You ought to likewise observe little and inconspicuous body sensations, for example, an itch or shivering. Try not to pass judgment on the senses. Instead, permit them to pass. It would help if you observed all emotions occurring in all aspects of your body, from your head to the toe.

Sensory

You should also note the sensory sensations such as the sights, sounds, smells, touches, or taste. Give them names and let them pass without any judgment.

Emotions

You should also let your emotions manifest without suppressing or judging them. You should name your feelings in a steady and relaxed way, such as "joy, anger, happiness."

Cravings and urges

You should let your cravings for addictive substances or behaviors to be present. Allow them to pass without judgment. Take a conscious mental note of how your body feels when the specific cravings enter.

How to Incorporate Mindfulness into Your Daily Life?

Mindfulness can be practiced anywhere and at any time of the day. No law limits mindfulness to sitting on a cushion.

You can incorporate the essential techniques of mindfulness into your everyday activities and tasks. Such events provide a lot of opportunities for you to carry out your mindfulness practice. You can cultivate mindfulness in your daily routine through some of the following practices:

While Washing Dishes

When you are busy doing the dishes, you hardly get any distractions from everyone else. The fact that you get little distractions when doing the dishes offers you an excellent opportunity to try some mindfulness.

As you clean your dishes and kitchen, you should train your mind to focus on the physical activity, making a note of the warm water on your hand, the sound of the clanking utensils, and the sound of the running water. All these activities and their accompanying sensations will help your mind focus on the present.

Brushing Your Teeth

You brush your teeth daily, sometimes more than twice each day. This could offer you an excellent opportunity to practice mindfulness meditation. Take note of the brush in your hand, the feet on the ground, and how your arm moves up and down as you undertake your brushing.

Driving

It is relatively easy to let your mind wander off when you are driving, but you should use your mindfulness power to anchor your thoughts to the present, focusing on the inside of your car. You can start by turning off your car radio or putting on some cool, soothing music. Then gently bring back your mind to the present, paying attention to where you are and what you are experiencing.

Exercising

You can practice mindfulness while atop your treadmill. Just focus on your breathing and where your feet are in space as you work on your treadmill. Pay close attention to the way you take in and out your breath. Notice how the pattern your legs create as your feet hit the mill or the ground.

CHAPTER 12:

Benefits of Intuitive Eating

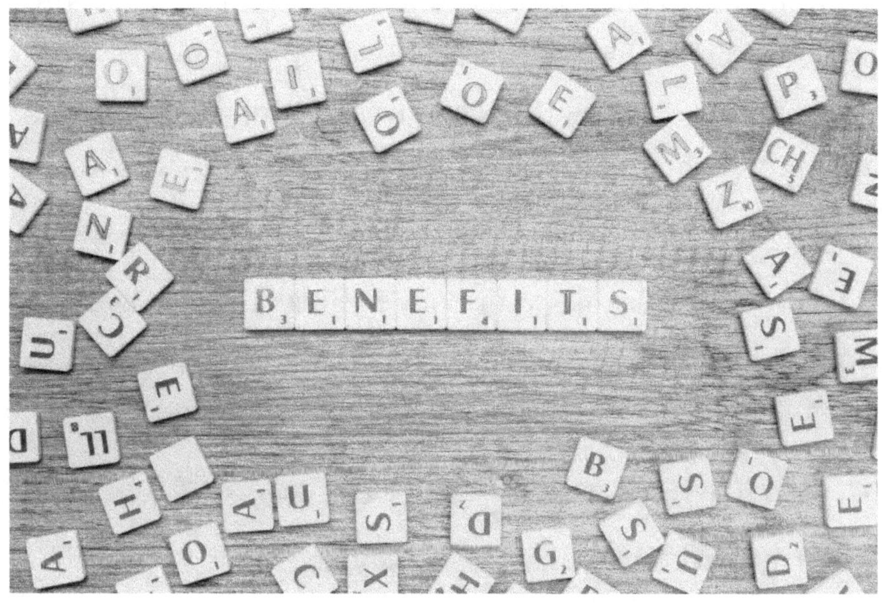

Intuitive eating isn't intended for weight reduction. Sadly, there might be dietitians, mentors, and different experts that sell intuitive eating as a diet, which runs counter to the thought altogether. The objective of intuitive eating is improving your association with food. This incorporates building more beneficial food practices and making an effort not to control the scale. That being stated, pretty much everyone experiencing the way toward figuring out how to be an intuitive eater needs to get thinner—else, they'd as of now be intuitive eaters!

Intuitive eating enables your body to break the diet cycle and sink into its regular set point weight territory. This might be lower, higher, or a similar weight you are at present.

How Intuitive Eating Plays a Role in Healthy Living and Shopping Lifestyle:

Intuitive eating guides our lives inside and out. It creates such a lot of opportunity and straightforwardness by not stressing over what I will eat or when I will eat it. I stream with what my body guides me to eat, and when it guides me to it eat-and with that, it creates opportunity inside my relationship in my body and how I feel about myself. I am more advantageous and more adjusted than I have ever been in my body, and I can say that I love my body and this vessel that I am carrying on with this life in.

This move-in my association with my body, food, and general surroundings is an immediate consequence of my otherworldly voyage.

The most significant thing is not to stress over the 'right' or 'wrong' choice, and instead to distinguish how you are feeling and where in your body you think it is the goal you aren't eating to keep away from concealing feelings. That way, you're eating decisions are simpler to make since they aren't enveloped with your passing feelings.

There is such a lot of opportunity and facilitate that shows up when you interface with and pursue your instinct. Shopping for food turns out to be, to a lesser degree, a task or a problem and increasingly an action of happiness and articulation. To have the option to purchase what looks, sounds, and scents great (offers to the faculties) and believe my instinct as far as what I will cook and create each day/week. It also makes the creation procedure progressively fun since you don't feel adhered to pursuing a formula or dinner plan. Once more, there is an opportunity. Shopping for food is only an expansion of that and part of the creation procedure (where motivation comes in).

Indeed, there might, in any case, be times when you don't feel like shopping for food or preparing; however, in those minutes, you aren't hung up on it. The dread of settling on a wrong choice or eating inappropriate food vanishes. Intuitive eating isn't about control and dread; it is about the stream and following what feels better (from a space of instinct, not damage or self-hurt).You are beginning the adventure of understanding what foods reverberate with your body and what doesn't-interfaces with the act of enthusiastic mindfulness. On the off chance that we shut ourselves off from feeling our feelings, at that point, we are additionally closing down our capacity to feel different sensations. Consider it like this-your body is sending you the flag of what feels better and what doesn't; however, you have unplugged the wire association between the inclination, and you are accepting and being informed of the disposition. Having an essential comprehension of sustenance is a great spot to start teaching oneself and acclimate oneself with specific establishments of pure sciences. From that point, it truly is an act of backing off and carrying your attention to how you feel during and after eating. At whatever point you notice examples of side effects, you should investigate. What musings did you see, how could you feel, what was going on around then? A great deal of our food and eating practices/designs have been adapted and created quite a while prior and requires bringing our cognizance again into that space to develop progressive movements. The most significant piece of this procedure is to curry sympathy with you and practice non-judgment.

The diet culture is a finished square to instinct. It is established in dread, and control-and expels the opportunity to interface with how you feel or what your body wants. The diet culture mirrors the longing to change and control the body instead of helping it and work with it. It is tied in with stifling the body's direction framework (through control), which expels you further away from your instinct and the capacity to interface with your intuition through your body's informing structure. The greatest thing to perceive is that your body is profoundly insightful and realizes what to do-the more that you work with it and backing (and trust it)- the more joyful you will feel. At whatever point we hop onto a pattern, it is imperative to associate with what feels better (and inquire whether this pattern genuinely impacts you or on the off chance that you are merely doing it since others are, and their outcomes entice you). A great spot to ground yourself in what your intuitive direction is, is to ask yourself, "What feels useful for your spirit?"

The Health Benefits of Intuitive Eating

Improvement in Digestion:

- Two of the fundamental precepts of intuitive eating are to:

- Eat just when you're ravenous,

- Eat until you're fulfilled, not stuffed.

- Rehearsing both of these propensities can help improve your assimilation in various manners.

For one, eating just when you're genuinely hungry gives your stomach related framework time to discharge your stomach from your last supper. This may appear no major ordeal, and however, when you continue eating each couple of hours and not enabling your food to process, your framework can undoubtedly move toward becoming exhausted. Your stomach needs to consistently siphon out chemicals and acids to help digest your food, while your liver is ceaselessly being attempted to channel poisons and condensation fat.

Additionally, eating until you're full at each feast can shield your assimilation from running comfortably. You're basically "Backing up" your framework by pouring undigested food over half-processed food, which may make you experience acid reflux, stoppage, or any number of stomach related issues.

Rehearsing body mindfulness, eating just until you're fulfilled, and not eating between suppers except if you're eager gives your stomach related framework a rest with the goal that it's completely prepared to deal with your dinner.

There Is No Room for Stress:

Studies have demonstrated that intuitive eaters not just appreciate a more lovely enthusiastic state than dieters, yet additionally experience enhancements in despair, nervousness, negative self-talk, and general mental prosperity when they change to eating intuitively.

The explanation behind this decrease in pressure may originate from how you get the chance to concentrate more on making the most of your food instead of dissecting it when you eat intuitively. You additionally remove yourself from the outlook of, "I can't have that since I have to get thinner," or "I can't have carbs because I'm fat."

These sorts of responses to food put a heap of weight at the forefront of your thoughts and body, so it's no big surprise you feel better when you let them go!

A Possibility to Aid Weight Loss:

Studies have likewise indicated that intuitive eaters have lower weight records (BMIs) than dieters. One of the significant purposes behind this could be that intuitive eating is anything but difficult to adhere to (not at all like trend diets), which can prompt long haul weight reduction.

When you eat intuitively, you also figure out how to regard a satiety flag that discloses to you when you're fulfilled versus only eating for eating. This outcome in a natural, ideal calorie balance could prompt weight reduction on the off chance you've been overeating by disregarding yearning signs.

Intuitive eating lessens feelings of anxiety can likewise assume a job since a lot of the pressure hormone cortisol can cause fat addition.

High Self-Esteem:

Notwithstanding improving eating examples and nervousness levels, contemplates have additionally demonstrated that rehearsing intuitive eating develops confidence.

For example, members in a single report experienced more acknowledgments of their bodies and less mental pain concerning their bodies. They were additionally ready to relinquish "Unfortunate weight control practices."

By improving your confidence, it's just typical that different parts of your life will improve too. At the point when you're concentrating less on not being "Sufficient" and more on tolerating yourself, you'll generally encounter less nervousness and have an increasingly inspirational point of view. Thus, this can prompt many open doors at work and enhancements in your connections.

A Decent Improvement in Body Awareness:

Monitoring your body and what it's motioning to you is critical with regards to keeping up your wellbeing. On the off chance that you listen intently, your body will offer you inconspicuous hints that something isn't right, enabling you to give it what it needs before it turns into a significant issue.

Take, for instance, indications of supplement inadequacies. Numerous individuals are so separated from their bodies that they don't see hidden signs of a supplement insufficiency, similar to an absence of vitality or shivering in their grasp and feet. When they understand, the inadequacy has turned out to be dangerous to such an extent that they need to go to the specialist to get it dealt with.

Intuitive eating is tied in with connecting with your body's sign of craving and satiety. Be that as it may, you'll begin to be hyper-mindful of different signs your body is emitting when you start focusing on these signs. This will enable you to be in line with what you need consistently, so you can deal with it before it turns into an all-out issue

CHAPTER 13:

Gastric band hypnosis

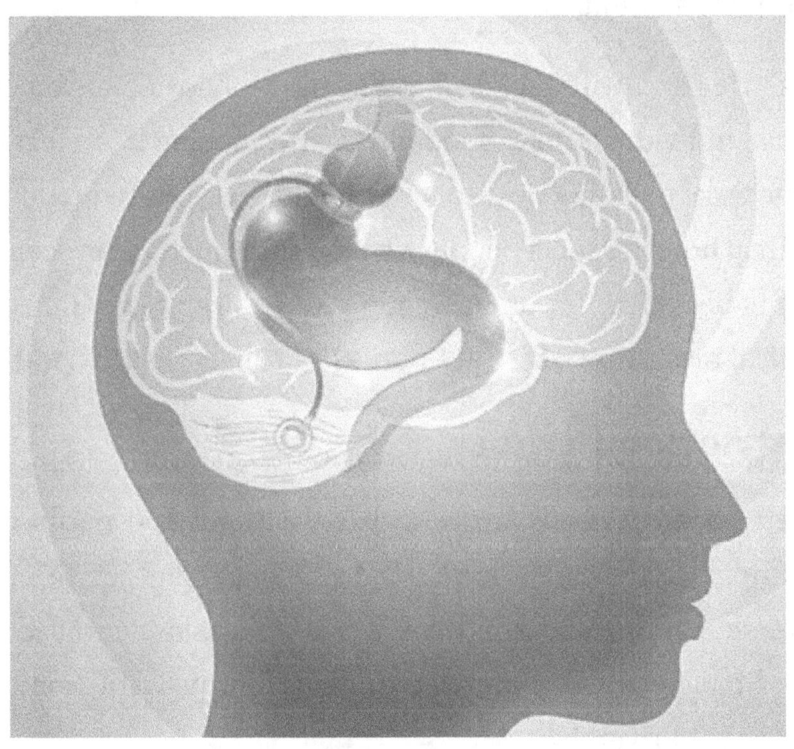

A stomach band is a silicone flexible apparatus utilized in weight reduction in medical procedures. To create a modest pack over the gadget, the band is put around the belly's upper part. This restrains the amount of sustenance that can be put away in the stomach area, making eating enormous amounts hard.

A gastric band will likely constrain the amount of sustenance that an individual can expend physically, making them feel full in the wake of eating next to no to advance weight reduction. It is a final hotel for most people who have this medical procedure after endeavoring for other weight reduction systems. Like any medical procedure, there are perils in fitting a gastric band.

Gastric Band Trance

Gastric band trance can be utilized without the perils that accompany medical procedures to help people get thinner. Numerous trance specialists use a two-dimensional procedure. The first hope to characterize your enthusiastic eating's underlying driver.

Utilizing trance, the specialist can urge you to recall long-overlooked nourishment related encounters that may now influence you subliminally. Before performing gastric band hypnotherapy, tending to and perceiving any unfortunate reasoning, examples concerning sustenance can help.

Next, the trance specialist will play out the treatment of the virtual stomach band. The technique is proposed to recommend that you had an activity to embed a gastric band at a subliminal stage. The objective is to cause your body to respond to this proposition by making you feel quicker as though you had an actual medical procedure.

How it Functions

How gastric band spellbinding works using unwinding a trance specialist techniques will get you a trance condition. Your subliminal is progressively open to proposal in this casual state. Trance inducers are making proposals to your intuitive at this stage. With hypnotherapy of the gastric band, this suggestion is that you have joined a physical band.

The psyche is solid, so your conduct will change as needs be on the off chance that you are subliminal that acknowledges these proposals. More often than not, alongside the virtual gastric band's' fitting,' proposals will be created about trust and conduct to help you focus on this way of life move.

Numerous specialists will likewise encourage strategies for self-mesmerizing so you can improve your activity after the session. It is regularly prescribed to instruct yourself on nourishment and exercise to help physical wellbeing and prosperity.

The Process

Your first subliminal specialist session will likely be a unique counsel to talk about what you would like to get from hypnotherapy. This is an opportunity to talk about any past endeavors at weight reduction, eating rehearses, medical issues, and generally speaking, nourishment frame of mind. This information will furnish the advisor with a clearer idea of what will help and whether to think about some other treatment methods.

The activity itself is expected to imitate the gastric band's medical procedure to help your subliminal think it has happened. Numerous subliminal specialists will incorporate the sounds and scents of a working performance center to make the experience increasingly true. Your specialist will begin by carrying you to a condition of profound unwinding, otherwise called entrancing. You'll be aware of what's happening, and you'll generally be in order.

The specialist will address you through the system once you're sleep-inducing. They will explain bit by bit what is happening in a medical procedure, from being put under a sedative to making the primary entry point, fitting the band itself, and sewing the cut. A working auditorium's sounds and scents will improve the experience to persuade your inner mind that what is said is transpiring.

As expressed before, different proposals to improve self-assurance might be incorporated during the activity. Endless supply of the system, your trance inducer may show you a few strategies for self-spellbinding to help you stay at home on the track.

Some subliminal specialists will approach you to return for follow-up arrangements to screen the virtual band's accomplishment and roll out any improvements. When people also fit the physical band, proceeding with hypnotherapy sessions as a feature of long-term weight management, the board plan might be valuable for a few. This empowers the subliminal specialist to work with you to handle the hidden sustenance and confidence issues.

How am I going to feel afterward?

The general objective of the gastric band is to encourage a more beneficial nourishment association. If your subliminal thinks you have a gastric band fitted, your stomach will believe it's lower. This, thus, makes your mind send messages that, in the wake of devouring less nourishment, you are finished.

Perceiving when you are physically finished can be hard for the individuals who gorge. At times we eat only for taste (or comfort), overlooking whether we are physically hungry or not. In developing smart dieting, figuring out how to perceive the physical vibes of being ravenous and finished is helpful.

In contrast to gastric band medical procedures, there are no physical symptoms in the virtual gastric band. The whole medical procedure may trigger the reflux of queasiness, regurgitating, and corrosive, for a few. Since the gastric band's mesmerizing is not a physical technique, it won't trigger such side effects.

The activity ought to be a charming and loosening up understanding, with most people revealing from entrancing an impression of quiet.

Is it going to work for me?

For the individuals who first attempt hypnotherapy, a well-known issue is - is it getting down to business for me? It is anything but a simple circumstance of yes or no, lamentably; it's mostly up to you. Hypnotherapy empowers people with an assortment of issues. However, it is instrumental in evolving propensities. Hence, helping people make excellent eating practices and shedding pounds is frequently viable. Like some other weight reduction plot, be that as it may, it will include your full commitment.

If you think simultaneously and your specialist, you're bound to get what you need from gastric band hypnotherapy. It is indispensable to be agreeable and to confide in your subliminal specialist. In this manner, it is prescribed that you require significant investment in your district to examine subliminal specialists and discover progressively about them, how they work, and what their aptitudes involve. Before the strategy, you can mastermind to meet them to ensure you are alright with them.

In case you're devoted to changing your way of life, think the methodology, and trust your subliminal specialist, the mesmerizing of the gastric band should work for you.

Using Hypnosis to Control Food Portions

Portion control can assume an amazing job in achieving your objectives for wellbeing and weight. You may, as of now, eat all the right sustenance and practice appropriately. In any case, in case regardless you're conveying overabundance weight, it may be because you're merely expending excessively. Control of segments can make a huge distinction.

Excellent portion control won't just thin you down; it will give you more vitality. Eating the right amount will suggest that your body needs to work more enthusiastically to process superfluous surplus nourishment.

Regarding getting your eating regimen right and shedding surplus fat, the amount is as fundamental as quality. If you have to get thinner, a lot of a decent thing can truly be terrible for you. However, knowing how, when, and the amount to cut so you can truly begin seeing some improvement in accomplishing your weight targets can be troublesome.

Why is Portion control so Hard to Achieve?

Propensity controls our lives substantially more than we understand. We eat because it's an ideal opportunity to eat (even though you had a nibble simply 30 minutes prior).

We're gorging out of good manners, or not having any desire to' squander' what's on our plate, or because we're so used to being full that we've overlooked how to perceive when we've had enough.

Some good judgment things can enable you to control the size of the bit:

- You can eat all the more gradually intentionally. This offers your stomach the chance to enlist its totality in your cerebrum and mood killer your hunger.

- You can begin your supper with soup-it very well may be fulfilling to have a low-calorie soup and enable you to feel cheerful for your fundamental course with a lot of little parts.

- You can utilize the old stunt of the little plate-so you need to eat littler segments truly.

- You can stay away from smorgasbords

Hypnosis is an incredible asset for controlling portions.

In any case, extraordinary as all the exhortation above maybe, despite everything, you have to conquer propensity and impulse, which is the place spellbinding can help. Nourishment is fuel, and the correct quality and amount of fuel are required. Envision attempting to place more fuel when it's full in your vehicle. It's simply not appearing well and good.

Portion control will take you to a profoundly loosened upstate and rapidly train your oblivious personality to intuitively realize when to disregard overabundance sustenance and make your assimilation considerably more agreeable. You will rediscover the joy of being tuned in to the dietary necessities of your own body.

The Power of the Gastric Band

A renowned and dramatic case of hypnotic power to influence our bodies directly is in the emergency treatment of burns. A few doctors have used hypnotic to accelerate and improve the recuperating of extreme injuries and help reduce the excruciating pains for his patients. If somebody is seriously burnt, there will be damage to the tissue, and the body reacts with inflammation. The patients are hypnotized to forestall the soreness. His patients heal quite rapidly and with less scarring.

There are a lot more instances of how the mind can directly and physically influence the body. We realize that chronic stress can cause stomach ulcers, and a psychological shock can turn somebody's hair into a grey color overnight. In any case, I especially like this aspect of hypnotism because it is an archived case of how the mind influences the body positively and medically. It will be somewhat of a miraculous event if the body can get into a hypnotic state that can cause significant physical changes in your body. Hypnotic trance without anyone else has a profound physiological effect. The most immediate effect is that subjects discover it deeply relaxing. Interestingly, the most widely recognized perception that my customers report after I have seen them—regardless of what we have been dealing with—is that their loved ones tell them they look more youthful.

Cybernetic Loop

Your brain and body are in constant correspondence in a cybernetic loop: they continually influence one another. As the mind unwinds in a trance, so too does the body. When the body unwinds, it feels good, and it sends that message to the brain, which thus feels healthier and unwinds much more. This procedure decreases stress and makes more energy accessible to the immune system of the body. It is essential to take note that the remedial effects of hypnotics don't require tricks or amnesia. For example, burns patients realize they have been burnt, so they don't need to deny the glaring evidence of how burnt parts of their bodies are. He practically hypnotizes them and requests that they envision cool, comfortable sensations over the burnt area. That imaginative activity changes their body's response to the burns.

The enzymes that cause inflammation are not released, and accordingly, the burn doesn't advance to a more elevated level of damage, and there is reduced pain during the healing process.

Using hypnotic and imagery, a doctor can get his patients' bodies to do things that are totally outside their conscious control. Willpower won't make these sorts of changes, but the creative mind is more grounded than the will. By using hypnotic and imagery to talk to the conscious mind, we can have a physiological effect in as little as 20 minutes

One and a half days after, the eczema was gone. With hypnotic, we can enormously enhance the effect of the mind. When we fit your hypnotic gastric band, we use the same strategy of hypnotic correspondence to the conscious mind. We communicate to the brain with distinctive imagery. The brain alters your body's responses, changing your physical response to food, so your stomach is constricted, and you feel truly full after only a few.

Visualization Is Easier Than You Think

The hypnotic we use to make your gastric band uses "visualization" and "influence loaded imager." Visualization is the creation of pictures in your mind. We would all be able to do it. It is an interesting part of the reasoning. For instance, think about your front door and ask yourself which side the lock is on. To address that question, you see an image in your mind's eye. It doesn't make a difference at all how reasonable or bright the image is, it is only how your mind works, and you see as much as you have to see. Influence loaded imagery is the psychological term for genuinely significant pictures. In this process, we use pictures in the mind's eye that have emotional significance.

Although hypnotic recommendations are incredible, they are dramatically upgraded by ground-breaking images when communicating directly to the body. For instance, you will be unable to accelerate your heart just by telling it to beat faster. Still, if you envision remaining on a railroad line and seeing a train surging towards you, your heart accelerates pretty quickly. Your body overreacts to clear, meaningful pictures.

It doesn't make a difference whether you are listening intentionally; your conscious mind will hear all it needs to recreate the real band, in a similar way that a clear image of a moving toward train rushing towards your influences your pulse rate. You do not have to hold the pictures of the operational procedures in your conscious mind because you are anesthetized and unconscious during an activity. Notwithstanding what you intentionally recollect, underneath the hypnotic anesthesia, your conscious mind uses this information and imagery to introduce your gastric band in the right spot.

Forms of Gastric Banding Procedures Used in Weight Reduction Hypnotherapy

Sleeve gastrectomy

This operation requires cutting half of a person's stomach, usually the size of a banana, to leave behind space. It will not be reversed once this portion of the stomach is cut away. This can sound like one of the more severe forms of gastric band operation, and it also poses several complications due to its degree of extremity. It does not sound worth it. However, it has been one of the more common procedures used in surgery as a restricting way of suppressing a patient's desire. For those who struggle with obesity, it is beneficial. As per medical experts, it has a reasonable performance rate and relatively few risks. Those who received the surgery suffered a reduction of up to 50% of their overall weight, which is quite a lot for those with obesity.

For others who struggle with compulsive eating problems, including binge eating, it is similarly effective.

A physician will make either a very wide or a pair of minor incisions in the abdomen as you get the surgery performed. It can take up to six weeks to heal from this operation physically.

Vertical banded gastroplasty

This gastric band treatment, commonly known as VBG, includes the same band positioned across the stomach during the sleeve gastrostomy. To shape a tight pouch, the stomach is then fastened above the band, which shrinks the gut in some manner to achieve the same results. Compared to several other forms of weight reduction treatment, the treatment has been recognized as a good one to reduce weight. While it might sound like a less complicated operation relative to a sleeve gastrostomy, it has a higher complication risk. This is why it is found much less prevalent. As of today, this unique gastric band operation is conducted by just 5% of bariatric specialists. Nevertheless, it is renowned for delivering outcomes and can also be used without hypnotherapy problems to achieve comparable effects.

Mixed Surgery (Restrictive and Malabsorptive)

A key feature in certain forms of weight reduction surgery is this method of gastric band operation. It is most generally referred to as a gastric bypass, which is conducted first, preceding all weight reduction procedures. It also contains stomach stapling and makes an intestinal form down your stomach. This is required to guarantee that the patient eats less food in conjunction with malabsorptive surgery, pointed to as a restrictive mixed procedure, ensuring that the body eats less food.

Everything You Need to Understand Regarding Gastric-Band Hypnotic Therapy

You may want to suggest doing the hypnotherapy component if you're unsure if the gastric band procedure is appropriate for you. Hypnotherapy is the ideal solution, as compared to an operation that has several risks, is 100 percent safer and, therefore, far more accessible. It has a performance rate of over 90 percent in patients, which is why more individuals choose it over gastric band procedure. Because you can do so in the safety of your own house as well, you don't have to think about the costs involved. Overall, it acts as a very easy way to tone down, decreasing the waste in nature. Again, no physical operation requiring intervention is used in hypnosis. It is a safe choice that lets you reach where you want to utilize creative and modern technologies. The hypnotherapy session includes visualizing the placing of a synthetic gastric band over your stomach that helps you to get the same feeling as you might initially have throughout surgery, but without the pain, unnecessary costs, and annoyance.

The result is that you feel like you are starving for longer stretches, need fewer calories, and feel whole, even though you have just consumed half of your regular-sized meal. This would also help you make better decisions and realize that a far better food experience than you presently have can be established. If you're curious if hypnotherapy for the gastric band would function for you, you should question whether you have the creativity to help your session. Everybody has an image now, of course, but is yours realistic enough? If you can shut your eyes and visualize staring at something that's not actually in front of you, then spend time reflecting on that, so you can effectively achieve so by gastric band hypnotherapy. Before you start something, it's natural to consider that it will struggle if it isn't adapted to you directly. Visual gastric band hypnosis will, however, provide emotional relief for you. This promotes your priorities, including weight reduction and improvement of fitness. When you invest time engaged in it, you can realize that you will accomplish whatever you put your purpose on. You will subconsciously erase your cravings, eliminate all detrimental and mental tension, as well as experiences that are part of your mental eating habit. Because impulsiveness forms a large amount of gaining weight, you can realize that it can be eliminated from your conscious mind and help any person willing to pursue it by hypnotherapy. As per a clinical report undertaken in the U.K., gastric band hypnotherapy has a 95% effective rate among patients. This analysis also found that certain patients would be willing to embrace and excel in hypnotherapy. Still, if they are not accessible to the experience, they will not find it useful. For a hypnotherapist's words to take action, individuals who are so cut off from fresh concepts, including hypnotherapy, sometimes made out to be a harmful activity by the uneducated, would not relax properly.

You'll know how it succeeds after only one hypnotherapy session since it is expected to start functioning after just one session. That is why all shouldn't get hypnotherapy. It is only recommended to someone prepared to shift their attitudes about food. It is called pointless if you do not trust it or bring you to where you want to go on your path towards weight reduction. Only after you have completed an appraisal will the expense of gastric band hypnotherapy services with a licensed hypnotherapist be determined. Energy stimulation strategies are often learned during these appointments and can also support any patient encounter with fear, frustration, tension, and all other harmful emotions.

CHAPTER 14:

Understanding the power of belief

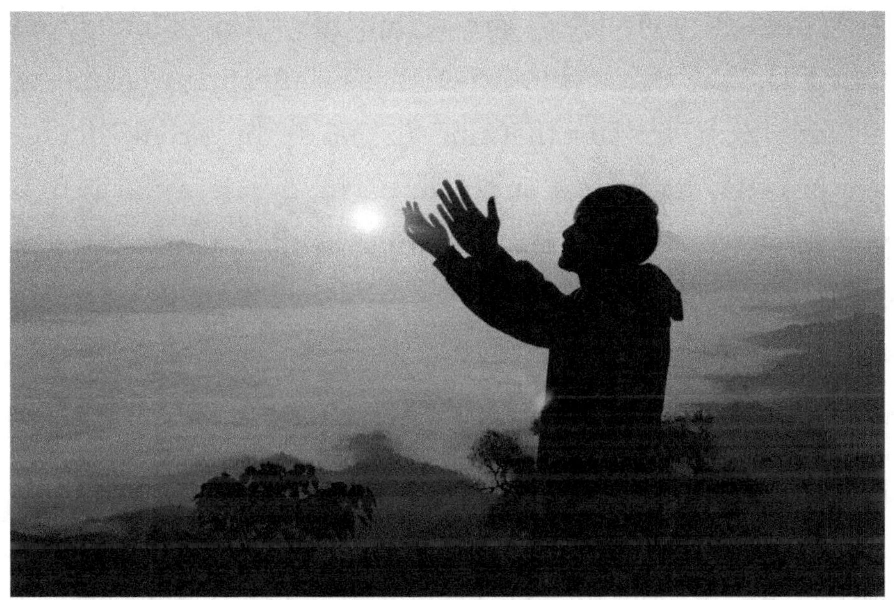

Belief and Believing

Beliefs are the thoughts valid to you. They may need not to be scientifically proven to realize them to be real for you. If you are aware of it or not, your movements, both conscious and subconscious, are functions of your beliefs. Even though your ideals are within the form of mind and thoughts, they shape your experience by affecting your moves in lifestyles. If you trust that animals make proper companions, you probably have a cat or dog or parrot or a ferret or two. If you agree with that coffee to continue with your conscious at night, you probably do no longer drink espresso before going to bed.

The electricity of believing helps you to affect your body in ways that might seem astounding. Placebo responses, where people reply to an inert substance as though it were the proper medicine, are not unusual examples of how we experience beliefs inside the body. If a person, in reality, believes that he will get well while taking a particular medicine, it will show up whether the tablet contains a remedy or is, without a doubt, inert. Identically, if someone without a doubt believes that he can achieve excessive grades in college, it'll appear. If someone believes that he can gain his best weight, it will manifest.

Remember your make-accept as real with games as a child. Your capacity to faux is just as sturdy now as while you had been very young. It can be a touch rusty, and you may want a bit of practice. However, while you allow yourself to be fake and believe in what you're pretending, you will find a powerful tool. You will discover that this is a wonderfully effective way to deliver your intentions, the ones with messages of what you need, to all the cells and tissues and organs of your body, which reply by bringing that purpose into reality for you.

We can't say this enough: thoughts are things. The thoughts, the pictures, and thoughts you put in your mind emerge as the messages your self-hypnosis conveys to your mind-body turn your ideal body into a truth. Pretending is choosing what to consider and turning into absorbed into one's ideas. Just as a magnifying glass can consciousness rays of sunlight, you could awareness your mental power to make your thoughts, ideas ideal for your shape.

Belief and Thinking

Whether you are mindful of it or perhaps not, your conscious and unconscious activities are based on the values of yours. Although your opinions are available in the shape of thoughts and ideas, they develop the experience of yours by changing the life activities of yours. In case you think that pets create beautiful companions, you more than likely have a dog or maybe parrot or cat or even a ferret or perhaps 2. In case you think that coffee will keep you awake during the night, you most likely do not drink coffee before you go to sleep.

The ability of thinking enables you to affect your entire body in a way that may appear astonishing. Placebo answers, where folks respond to an inert chemical as if they were the right medicine, are typical examples of how beliefs have been experienced within the body. If an individual believes he will become well when carrying a specific treatment, it will take place if the pill includes drugs or is only perceptible. In precisely the same manner, if an individual believes he can attain high school levels, it will occur.

If an individual believes he can reach his ideal weight, then it is going to occur. Recall your chosen matches as a kid. Your capacity to feign is equally as powerful now as if you're young. It Might Be a little rusty, and you may require a bit of exercise, but when you allow yourself to feign and think about what you're pretending, you will see a powerful instrument.

You will find that this can be a superbly productive method to produce your aims, these messages of everything you would like, to everyone the cells and organs and tissues of the human body, which react by bringing that aim in reality for you. We cannot state this enough: ideas are things. The ideas, the images, and thoughts you set in your head become the messages that your self-hypnosis communicates into a mind-body, finally turning your ideal body into a truth. Pretending is picking what to think and getting absorbed in these thoughts.

As a magnifying glass may concentrate beams of the sun, you can focus your emotional energy to create your ideas, thoughts, and beliefs actual for your physique.

Expectation

You might not always get what you would like, but you do get what you expect. Expectations include the power of faith, and eventually, become the outcomes of what's considered. Here's a good illustration of how to "expect." Once you sat down to read this novel, you didn't analyze the seat or couch to check its ability to maintain your weight. You simply sat down without even considering it.

You did not have to Consider It because a piece of your convinced, and contains so much religion in the seat, which you "anticipated" it to maintain you. That's the best way to anticipate the ideal body weight you would like. Bearing this in mind, be cautious of everything you say to yourself and others, seeing your body weight expectations. "I gain weight through the holidays" "Last evening I ate two pieces of cake, and this morning I had been just two pounds heavier."

Mind-Body in Focus

Every one of the vital ingredients may create powerful results when concentrated inside the mind-body. But when these ingredients have been calibrated correctly inside the self-hypnosis procedure, their efficacy has still magnified a hundredfold. Self-hypnosis is a procedure for making your reality. You may think that sounds magic or too fantastic to be correct, but that's relative to what you've got to this stage in your life. These thoughts may be relatively fresh for you. Here's a good instance of this "comparative" character of fresh thoughts.

Imagine that you're supplied a personal jet that's beautifully equipped with luxury appointments and also a well-trained crew. It's a fantastic gift, and you also get to reveal this technology marvel to some people who have not ever seen anything like this. Let's suppose your pilot strikes you back in time to before December 17, 1903, when the Wright brothers declared their first flight in Kitty Hawk. You're happy to reveal this miracle of technology to the Wright brothers, who come to greet you personally. What could happen? Maybe they'd be scared and would not think it is possible to fly into a metallic bird. You can give them a ride, and they may opt to run out of you. Folks can reject or resist new ideas, even if they're lovely.

Your subconscious (mind-body) utilizes the combo of everything you need (inspiration), everything you think, and what you anticipate as a blueprint for actions. The outcomes are attained by your mind-body (unconscious), rather than by studying or thinking. If somebody reaches a cold surface she thinks is quite sexy, she can generate a blister or burn reaction. Conversely, an individual touching a scorching surface, believing it is cold, might not create a burn reaction. Individuals who walk across hot flashes while imagining they are cool might undergo thermal harm (some slight scorching around the bottoms of the feet); however, their immune system doesn't react with a burn (blistering, pain, etc.) since their heads inform their bodies the way to respond. Again, it's the orientation of three of those vital ingredients which makes it easy:

- Desiring to take action

- Thinking it possible

- Hoping to become successful

The truth goes through three phases. First, it's ridiculed. Second, it's violently opposed. Third, it's considered to be self-evident.

That is the trick to achievement. Your entire body carries your own beliefs. Your beliefs guide your activities, which then form your expertise. Some explain this procedure as creating your achievement or producing your expertise in life.

In our civilization, we view this clarified within the inspirational and positive emotional attitude literature. It may be understood in several regions of metaphysics. It is also possible to look back at the ancients and watch what is explained in the historical period's details.

An individual much wiser than we're mentioned, "It'll be done unto you based on your view." In the current era of integrative psychology and medicine, we predict it self-hypnosis or mind-body medication. There continue to be many scientific studies that demonstrate surprising consequences for pain management, wound healing, physical change, and a lot more health benefits than we thought possible.

Choosing Your Beliefs

You can pick your beliefs. You might decide to think what you find, in the feeling of "See it to believe it" or even "Seeing is believing" That is pretty simple to accomplish. You encounter something together with your perceptions, and that's a comfortable manner of picking whether it's believable or not. However, you might also opt to think about it and then watch it, which might require some exercise. Many men and women find it simpler to allow the world to tell them what's accurate or what to think. The T.V, newspapers, media, novels, teachers, and specialists bombard us with everything to consider. You grew up learning about the planet and yourself from several outside resources. It also led to a recognizable routine of discovering and observing information concerning the earth from yourself, and you decided which advice to create part of your belief system. It comprised belief about your physique. As an instance, as soon as your belly produces a sound noise, you feel that means you're hungry. Or you are feeling nauseous and think you're sick. Both are examples of noticed events: you discovered a link once and decided to consider it. From the Rapid Weight Loss Diet," we're suggesting that you just turn that clinic around for this thought: "Think it, and you'll see it" It follows that you choose what to think, then your entire body works on it as authentic and which makes it real on your adventure. Among the important messages we expect that you will receive from that book is your mind-body hears that you hear, what you say, all you presume, imagine, or picture in your head, and it can't tell the difference between what's actual and everything you envision. It behaves upon what you would like, thinks, and hope. Remember, these statements would enable you to experience the ideal weight you want: "I only look at food and gain weight" or even "I will eat my weight remains the same"? Indeed, the latter. However, that statement do you believe to be authentic for you? Again, it is going to be done unto you based on your view. We'll help you with the thoughts, speech, and graphics that invent practical hypnotic ideas, but you need complete control of what you opt to trust. As you browse the tips in this novel and discover the hypnotic suggestions provided through the trancework about the sound, you may have many options. We wholeheartedly invite you to opt to think about it. You will notice it on your own. Your subconscious (mind-body) can't tell the difference and act on which you pick either manner. Why don't you decide what you want?

The Power of Emotions

Few ideas and beliefs manifest themselves in your expertise. Just the ones which possess the ability of your emotions (feelings), together with your perception and your anticipation that something will occur, will manifest themselves.

Your emotions or emotions are a Kind of energy which affects this procedure for creation. In other words, whenever you've got a strong feeling of a belief, then it includes energy. This energy generates your expertise and further strengthens your expectations and beliefs. We're speaking about your ideas' collective energy, beliefs, preferences, and what exactly you would like.

The psychological energy supports what you would like and just how much you allow yourself to desire; it generates inspiration. It's possible to observe it is crucial to let yourself want something with a good feeling. If you blend feeling with desire, you enable the procedure you're putting into motion inside you. Ensure your feelings stay optimistic. You can determine when they're negative or positive regarding how they make you feel. It is simple.

Emotions that cause you to feel good are favorable, and feelings that cause you to feel awful are unfavorable. Maintain each of these energies confident by feeling great about your needing (want), faith, and expectations. If you've got negative thoughts and emotions, then they'll harm your motivation. If you've got positive ideas and feelings, then they will fortify your motivation. Ideas, beliefs, and expectations will be equal-opportunity energies. You're able to bring them and create negative or positive results and results. If you're negative, then expect adverse outcomes. If you're positive, anticipate positive effects. In this way, any notion, opinion, or expectation produces a positive or negative result. It is a no-brainer--if you need success, seek good energy from positive ideas and feelings. Charles talked a litany of unwanted words. "My job is overpowering.

I don't have any opportunity to do anything but grow from bed in the morning, drive into the workplace, and attempt to keep everyone happy. I get a headache just thinking about my life. I cannot possibly consider losing weight; it's not in the film." Guess what? Charles gets upset all of the time, and that he continues to lose excess weight, and he'll do so until he quit having negative words to describe his life.

Choosing Your Feelings

Your mind-body also calms your perception according to your inherent sense. Here's a good illustration. Let's suppose you wish to think about something which can allow you to realize your objective. You write an affirmation and start saying it to yourself. Affirmations are an excellent means to produce positive suggestions and customs. Speaking affirmations enables your ears to listen to your voice. It also is a method of picking your beliefs and strengthening them. For Instance, you might say that the affirmation, "I'm thinner and lighter now." However, what would you believe? If you "feel" that you weigh too much or believe the affirmation is false and inform yourself of the affirmation anyhow, there's a battle. Everything you are feeling is just another way your subconscious mind your perception or hold as correct. Your feelings must be in working with your affirmations along with your desires, beliefs, and preferences. Remember, emotions (feelings) are all energy. You could be asking, "But what if I do not think what I am telling myself?" Can it anyway. It's far better than focusing on the power of your own emotions, needs, and faith in a negative way.

The Law of Dominant Effect

There's essential legislation about hypnosis, Known as the Law of Dominant Effect. It informs us that anything that dominates our idea, whatever modulates our perception, is what our bodies will act upon. So, if 51% of your brain considers "A," and just 49% of your brain feels "B," you will have "A," precisely what most, or even the dominance, your ideas are. It usually means you don't need to have utterly fantastic beliefs; you merely need to have the benefit of your opinion concentrated on what you would like. Indeed this is a situation where "better is better."

Time Is on Your Side

You don't need to be worried about just how long some routines or programs happen to be operating on your subconscious or mind-body. They could change the moment you find what Has to Be adjusted or realigned, in Addition to when you make the intentional option to alter them. We'd want you to be aware of how your mind-body comprehends time.

You're conscious of the mechanical and linear dimension of time in days, minutes, hours, and seconds--that which we call "clock time." That's the way your conscious mind knows the dimension of time. Your unconscious, you're mind-body, just knows "today time," at which one moment can look like ten, or even ten minutes may look like you, or what's occurring in the "now." On your sleeping, you can undergo a fantasy happening in the area you lived as a young child, but with individuals who went to a high school, folks you may notice in tomorrow's scheduled assembly, and also the individual who took your purchase for lunch daily. All this may happen at the Exact Same time in your fantasy, as your subconscious love all Moment as "now."

Throughout your trance work, you may discover Dr. G. mention your subconscious may use the hypnotic suggestions together with pictures and thoughts of their future as if they've already happened.

Considering that most of the time is "now time" for your subconscious, you can correct, substitute, or make the suggestions and programs which you would like to "conduct" in you "now."

CHAPTER 15:

Deep sleep meditation

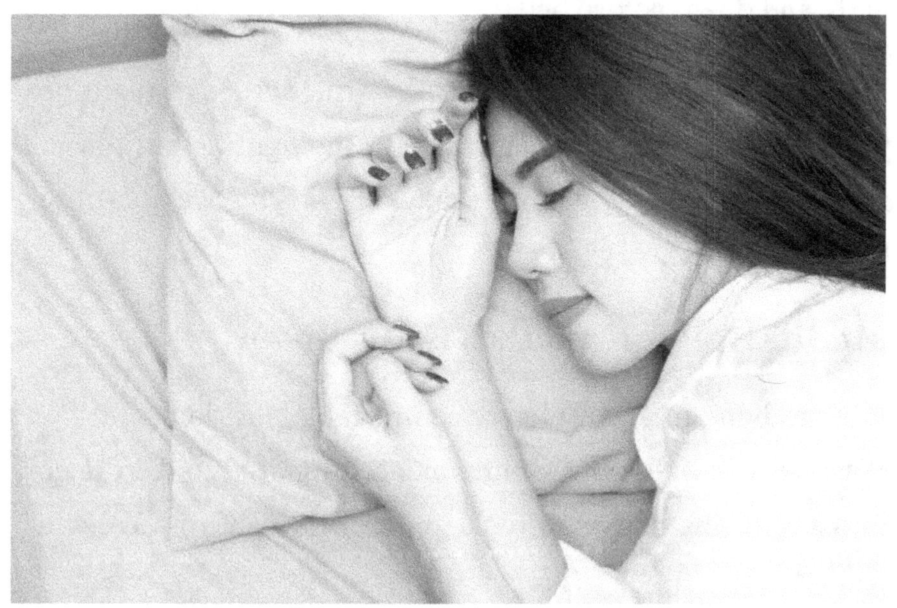

One of the best ways to relax and find the peace needed for better sleep is through a visualization technique. For this, you will want to ensure that you are in a completely relaxing and comfortable place. This reading will help you be more centered on the moment, alleviate anxiety, and wind down before bed.

Listen to it as you are falling asleep, whether it's at night or if you are simply taking a nap. Ensure the lighting is right and remove all other distractions that will keep you from becoming completely relaxed.

Meditation for a Full Night's Sleep

You are lying in a completely comfortable position right now. Your body is well-rested, and you are prepared to drift deeply into sleep. The deeper you sleep, the healthier you feel when you wake up.

Your eyes are closed, and the only thing that you are responsible for now is falling asleep. There isn't anything you should be worried about other than becoming well-rested. You are going to be able to do this through this guided meditation into another world.

It will be the transition between your waking life and a place where you will fall into a deep and heavy sleep. You are becoming more and more relaxed, ready to fall into a trance-like state where you can drift into a night of healthy sleep.

Start by counting down slowly. Use your breathing in fives to help you become more and more asleep.

Breathe in for ten, nine, eight, seven, six, and out for five, four, three, two, and one. Repeat this once more. Breathe in for ten, nine, eight, seven, six, and out for five, four, three, two, and one.

You are now more and more relaxed and prepared for a night of deep and heavy sleep. You are drifting away, faster and faster, deeper and deeper, closer and closer to a heavy sleep. You see nothing as you let your mind wander.

You are not fantasizing about anything. You are not worried about what has happened today or even farther back in your past. You are not afraid of what might be there going forward. You are not fearful of anything in the future that is causing you panic.

You are highly aware within this moment that everything will be OK. Nothing matters but your breathing and your relaxation. Everything in front of you is peaceful. You are filled with serenity, and you exude calmness. You only think about what is happening in the present moment where you are becoming more and more at peace.

Your mind is blank. You see nothing but black. You are fading faster and faster, deeper and deeper, further and further. You are getting close to being completely relaxed, but you are OK with sitting here peacefully right now.

You aren't rushing to sleep because you need to wind down before bed. You don't want to go to bed with anxious thoughts and have nightmares about the things you fear. The only thing you concern yourself with at this moment is getting friendly and relaxed before it's time to start to sleep.

You see nothing in front of you other than a small white light. That light becomes a bit bigger and bigger. As it grows, you start to see that you are inside a vehicle. You are laying on your bed. Everything around you is still there. Only when you look up, you see that there is a large open window, with several computers and wheels out in front of you.

You realize that you are in a spaceship floating peacefully through the sky. It is on auto-pilot, and there is nothing that you have to worry about as you are floating up in this spaceship. You look out above you and see that the night sky is more gorgeous than you ever could have imagined.

All that surrounds you is nothing but beauty. Bright stars are twinkling against a black backdrop. You can make out some of the planets. They are all different than you would ever have imagined. Some are bright purple, and others are blue. There are detailed swirls and stripes that you didn't know were there.

You relax and feel yourself floating up in this space. When you are here, everything seems so small. You still have problems back home on Earth, but they are so distant that they are almost real. Some issues make you feel as though the world is ending, but now that the entire universe is still doing fine, no matter what might be happening in your life. You are not concerned with any issues right now.

You are soaking up all that is around you. You are so far separated from Earth, and it's crazy to think about just how much space is out there for you to explore. You are relaxed, looking around. There are shooting stars all in the distance. There are floating rocks passing by your ship. You are floating around, feeling dreamier and dreamier.

You are passing over Earth again, getting close to going back home. You are going to be sent right back into your room, falling more heavily with each breath you take back into sleep. You are getting closer and closer to drifting away.

You pass over the earth and look down to see all of the beauty that exists. The green and blue swirl together, white clouds above that make such an interesting pattern. Everything below looks like a painting. It does not look real.

You get closer and closer, floating so delicately in your small space ship. The ride is not bumpy. It is not bothering you.

You are floating over the city now. You see random lights flicker on. It doesn't look like a map anymore, like when you are so high above.

You are looking down and seeing that gentle lights still flash here and there, but for the most part, the city is winding down. Everyone is drifting faster and faster to sleep. You are getting closer and closer to your home.

You see that everything is peaceful below you. The sun will rise again, and tomorrow will start. For now, the only thing you can do is prepare and rest for what might come.

You are more and more relaxed now, drifting further and further into sleep.

You are still focused on your breathing; it is becoming slower and slower. You are close to drifting away to sleep now.

When we reach one, you will drift off deep into sleep.

Sleep Well with Self-Hypnosis

This is going to be a thirty-minute guided hypnosis session to help you drift off into a deep and relaxing sleep. The most important thing to do while listening to this session is to keep an open mind. You must go with the flow, listen to my voice, and remember to breathe. Remember, it is not always possible to enter a light hypnotic state on the first try, but we will try as I guide you gently and smoothly into this state to fall asleep. Please bear in mind that you are not going to enter any sort of deep catatonic state. Nothing is going to be physically altered within the realm of your mind. The process of hypnosis and this guided meditation is exceptionally safe, and you are in control of it.

Now, I want you to get comfortable. Because you are trying to achieve deep sleep, you should be lying down, your head resting on your most comfortable pillow, and warmed by your softest blanket. Lie back and let your shoulders go slack, relaxing against the cushion of your bed. Gently close your eyes and release all the tension from your muscles. Release the tension in your arms, then your legs. Let go of the stress in your chest and your back. All of your body muscles begin to feel looser and looser, and your body is feeling light.

Recognize that this is a time for only you. You have set aside all of your day's activities and are ready to embrace a beautiful and peaceful sleep fully. Breathe in this moment of relaxation, where nothing else matters. There is only you in the warmth of your bed.

As you lay, I will ask you something very simple. In your mind's eye, imagination a kind of ruler or some sort of measuring device. Imagine something which can measure the depth of your relaxation. Imagine this ruler in front of your mind. Perhaps it is your favorite color, smooth with small painted tick marks and numbers.

Take a moment to notice where you are at your current level of relaxation, out of a scale of 100 down to 0 being your most relaxed state. Understand that there is no right or wrong measurement, to begin with. Explore your state, be honest with yourself as you measure your relaxation. What tensions do you still have left in your body? What anxieties, sadness, or pain still lingers? Very soon, you will increase your relaxation and melt away this negativity and drift off into a peaceful sleep.

Perhaps you are currently at a 60 on your scale of relaxation. Even though you may be lower down than that, imagine yourself moving the marker in front of you. With each deep breath, you slide the marker further down along this ruler closer and closer towards zero, towards immense relaxation. As you breathe and the marker slides down, you feel your muscles release in your arms, then your legs, your back relaxes, and your chest opens like a flower, welcoming in big and tranquil breaths.

You may be aware that your sense of relaxation has expanded inside of you. Perhaps down to 40 or 30. You see the marker slowly glide downwards along the scale. You feel that a wave of warmth has washed over you, and you are beginning to feel your whole body becoming engulfed in the warmth of peace. As you feel your body releasing its tension even more now, you feel calmer. You have now reached a ten on your scale, and gently, you take a deep breath through your nose. Let it fill your stomach until it is like to burst. Then release it.

You reach nine...You enter a peaceful, calm environment.

You reach eight...You can feel the warmth of the sun on your face. It is a reminder that you are loved.

You reach seven...Each sound that you hear, you do not deny. Instead, it lulls you further and deeper into a deep state of relaxation.

You reach six...You inhale through your nose and fill your belly. You inhale all of the good things the world has to offer.

You reach five...Gently, through your nose, you release your breath. You expel any negative feelings that remain.

You reach four...You feel your body becoming lighter. Your arms and legs feel weightless and free.

You reach three...You feel your chest brimming with warmth and light.

You reach two... You accept the peace that has enveloped you. This peace welcomes you into a deepening serenity as your mind quiets.

You reach one... You feel yourself drawn towards the warmth of peaceful sleep, so close you can almost graze it with your fingertips.

You reach zero... You feel a comfort deep within you that starts in your chest and radiates outwards like a blooming flower. This comfort fills you with security, and you remember that you are safe. You have released your worries and concerns, and in its place, there is warmth, light, and comfort.

Gently you are lulled by this wave of serenity. You feel yourself beginning to drift beyond zero, into a realm of warm colors. Billows of reds and pinks, yellows, and oranges undulate around you in soft embraces until you float down onto a plush, cool surface.

With only your fingertips, you detect that you have landed on a grassy field. Around you, you can smell the sweet fragrance of wildflowers that have populated this clearing. Your body and mind have quieted to listen to the soft rustle of the breeze through grass and flower petals, and you remember the beauty of the earth. You breathe in through your nose, a deep breath that fills your stomach. Through your nose, you slowly release it.

You recognize the warm colors from before, now painted in the sky. The reds fade into pinks seamlessly as though crafted by a painter's brush. The hues swirl into the setting sun and exude a warmth that you feel throughout your body. You exist in this space with only beauty. You live without concern for time or worry. There is only you in this space, and all of the tranquility it shares with you.

The pinks give way to magentas, then onto violets and dark blues. The sunsets and reveals an endless sky, sprinkled with thousands of twinkling stars. You see dustings of silver and purple in the sky. The bright sliver of the moon casts its beam upon you, cascading you in comfort.

Your muscles seem to melt, going slack, and welcoming sleep. The stars above you dance, twirling through the vast stretch of sky, but you are still. You allow this positive energy to enter your mind. It swells within you until you feel peace exuding from every pore. You have reached a depth of serenity that exists on the brink of sleep. Allow yourself to accept rest.

Underneath the moon, you accept rest. Soon, you begin to notice a new pleasing sensation that arrives at your arms and spreads to your legs and your back, your neck, and forehead. You recognize this sensation as sublime floating energy entering your body. You feel a delicate tingle throughout your body, ushering in lightness and calmness. This sensation is like soft white linen, cleansing you from the inside out. It is a warm touch of healing energy, love, and passion.

These soft vibrations rid you of tension. Anxieties are expelled. Sadness and fear no longer exist here. All of the excess stress is now dissolving entirely, turning into dust carried off by the wind. It is melting away under the power of this healing energy. In its place, there is safety and the knowledge that you are loved by whom you love. It is merely you, the stars, and the moon.

The lightness you feel swells as if tiny balloons are attached to different parts of your body. You feel your body beginning to rise and drift upwards in the direction of the stars. Peacefulness and serenity are lifting you higher into the air into the welcoming embrace of the expansive night sky. For a brief moment, you understand that you exist in the space between the earth and the sky, a realm that belongs to you and is safe from anxiety. You claim this realm as yours in which to dream. This is your dreamscape, where you float towards rest and sleep. Your realm is one of peace that connects the heavens with the ground. It is yours alone to govern, to allow only positive energy and love. You roam over the tops of trees, drift across the width of lakes, and coast above others, sleeping in their warm beds.

Your entire body now is floating higher and higher in this realm as you feel such joy inside as you realize you are now gliding through all of space. You are drifting and roaming here, no longer bound by gravity. You are now soaring like a hot air balloon, ascending higher and moving towards the infinity of this welcoming expansion. As you float, you are letting go of everything that you no longer need. You toss away unwanted negativity. You hold on to the comfort that peace grants you.

As you become just like the pure brilliance of the stars, a beautiful shining light, you feel your spirit break free, and finally, you can float out through the entire universe. You reach out further and further into the purest wisdom and the most loving embraces of all of the celestial beings surrounding you. They are calling you to rest, to dream, to sleep, to heal. You feel yourself realigning from within.

You feel yourself moving with tranquility and mindfulness, further and further. As you wade through the stars, you feel yourself gently feeling heavier. You understand that you are drifting towards rest.

You drift through the cosmos, feeling gravity's kind tug towards the ground. Gently you float towards the earth as a leaf falls from a tree, eager to meet its rest based below. You feel completely relaxed and slipping away into a restful sleep. Before you escape into your dreams, you return to your bed, where you are warm and protected. Your body softly nestles under the blankets, and your head snuggles into the pillow. You notice your arms and legs still feel weightless, and there is a residual warm vibration throughout, a pulsing that beseeches sleep. You happily oblige.

I am going to count down from five. When I reach one, you will fully embrace the peace that has engulfed you and lose yourself in sleep. You will feel yourself slipping into a calm and serene rest.

Five... You think of the night sky and its expansiveness. It melts away every remaining tension until your body and mind are relaxed. It is summoning your sleep.

Four... You feel the warmth of peace move from the top of your head and down your neck. It moves through your shoulders, radiates through your chest and stomach, and finally glazes over your legs.

Three... You feel your body become heavy, and you softly sink in a little deeper to your consciousness. You are safe and protected.

Two... You feel yourself drift away, like a leaf on a still pond. You float away quietly into the night.

One... You are now asleep, resting, and at peace.

Breathe in, breathe out. Breathe in, breathe out. When you wake, you will be refreshed and ready to take on the day. You will be prepared to conquer the stresses of your life now that you have conquered sleep.

CHAPTER 16:

A Lifelong Journey

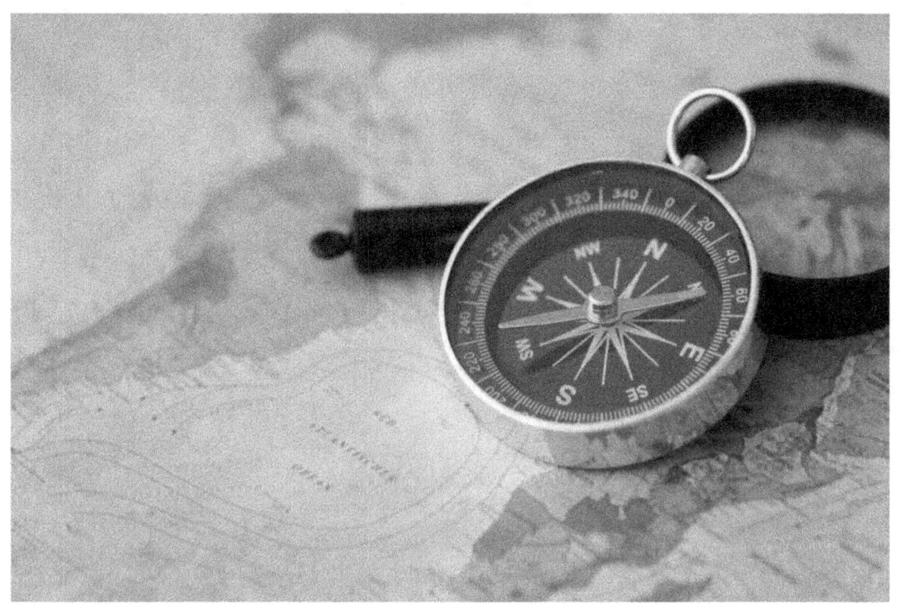

When we think about having to do something successfully, we often get caught up with the idea that we have to do things all at once. You have to pace yourself. If you're casually jogging instead of sprinting, then you're going to have a much lower chance of tripping and falling.

It will take just as long to change to a positive lifestyle as it took to get into a negative one. Unfortunately, we conditioned ourselves to think in a certain negative way. We often felt like we were not working toward our "success" or whatever we had defined it, as if we couldn't measure it in large tangible amounts. We have to start to look at the smaller things in life that can lead to success. Not everything has to be so big, so overdone. Instead, we can simply look at our jeans being a little loose on us as a massive milestone, rather than expecting to be able to fit into a much tinier size right away. Learn to take things in smaller amounts, and after a while, you will see the bigger picture.

We have to focus on methods that we can measure our success. Often, people will do this with numbers. They will hop on a scale, pull out a tape measure for their waste, or look at how quickly they might have been able to lose a certain amount of weight. None of this matter! You have to instead focus on the little milestones and how you feel overall. Sometimes, we measure success too much in ways that we think we can quantify. Everyone's journey will look different, including the victories we manage to make along the way.

You did your best; that's something that should be rewarded. If you can say that you honestly tried, then you should feel proud. You might not have gotten exactly what you wanted out of an individual situation, but you should still feel incredibly proud that you attempted something without giving up. As you move along your journey, your successes can get easier to measure, and you will also have larger goals. That is fine, though, because you will have the tools needed to achieve those more challenging goals.

CHAPTER 17:

Positive affirmations

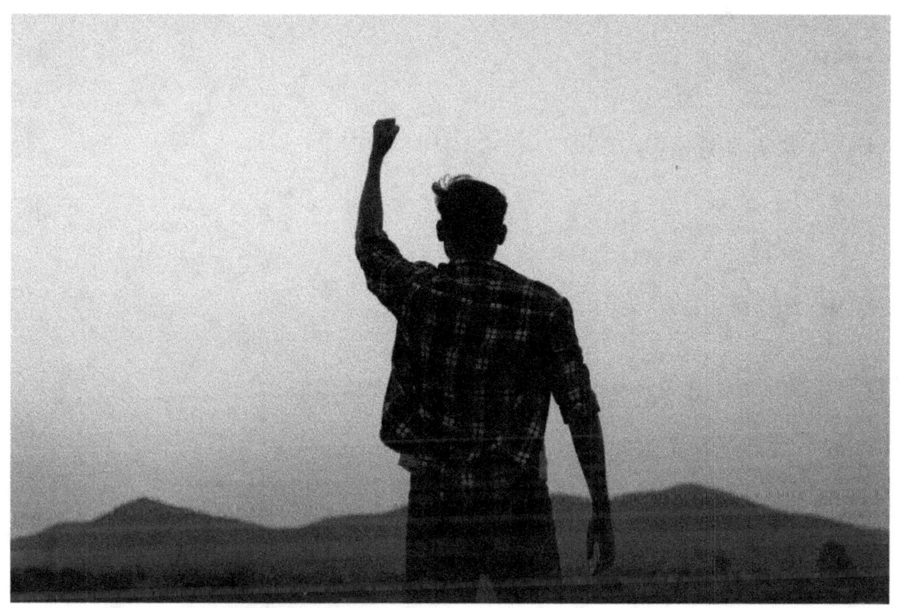

Thanks to my creator and everyone in my life.

I am grateful for all the bounty that I already enjoy

Every day I grow energetically and vibrantly

I only give my body the necessary nutritious food

My body is my temple

You can always maintain a healthy weight

I deserve to enjoy perfect health

Act to be healthy

I respect my body and am willing to exercise

My body is beautiful and healthy

I choose healthy and nutritious foods

I like to exercise, and I do it frequently

Losing weight is easy and even fun

I have confidence in myself

I am now sure of myself

I feel confident to succeed

From day today, I am more and more confident

I am sure to reach my goal

I want to be a noble example

I believe in my value

I have the strength to realize my dreams

I am adorable

I trust my inner wisdom

Everything I do satisfies me deeply

I trust the process of life

I can free the past and forgive

No thought of the past limits me

I get ready to change and grow

I am safe in the Universe, and life loves me and supports me

With joy, I observe how life supports me abundantly and provides me with more goods than I can imagine.

Freedom is my divine right

I accept myself and create peace in my mind and my heart

I am a loved person, and I am safe.

Divine Intelligence continually guides me in achieving my goals

Fear is a simple emotion that cannot stop me from succeeding

Every step forward I make increases my strength

My hesitations give way to victory

I want to do it, and I can do it

I am capable of great things

There is no one more important than me

That I can handle it

With confidence, I can accomplish everything

I allow myself to have a lot of fun

I deserve to be seen, heard, and shine

I deserve love and respect

I choose to believe in myself

I allow myself to feel good about myself and trust myself

I reduce measures quickly and easily

I can maintain my ideal weight without any problems

My body feels light and in perfect health

I'm motivated to lose weight and stay

Every day I reduce measures and lose weight

I fulfill my weight loss goals

I lose weight every day, and I recover my perfect figure

I eat like a thin person

I treat my body with love and give it healthy food

I choose to feel good inside and out

I feed myself only until I am satisfied. I don't saturate my food body

I know how to choose my food in a balanced way.

I feed slowly and enjoy every bite.

I am the only one who can choose how I eat and how I want to see myself.

It is easy for me to control the amount of what I eat.

I learn to have habits that lead me to my ideal weight.

Being at my ideal weight makes me feel healthy and young.

My body is very grateful and quickly reflects all the care I have for him.

My body reflects my perfect health.

I feel better every day

Being at my ideal weight motivates me to do other things that I like.

The human body is moldable, and I am the () artist of my body.

Every day I eat with awareness.

I consume the calories needed to have an ideal weight and a healthy body.

Every day I like the way I feel.

My slender body makes me feel agile, light (and) and healthy at the same time.

I know how to calculate the portions my body needs to feel adequately satisfied.

I can achieve everything that I propose.

No one can do this for me. Only I can make the best version of me, inside and out.

I am an inspiration for other people.

I like how the clothes look on my slender body.

I am strong, physically, and mentally.

No one can get me out of my motivation for being a healthy and slender person.

Being at my ideal weight fills me with energy.

My metabolism is faster every day thanks to the food I eat.

I love my new lifestyle.

I am getting better and better.

I accept all the blessings of the universe.

Reality is created from my thoughts.

I decide to choose thoughts that will have a positive impact on my life.

I am open to all new experiences of life.

I am free to think about what I want.

I will achieve great things.

I will be the best to accomplish this task.

I value myself because I am the right person.

I have full possession of my means.

I hide all the negative things that I cannot change.

I love myself a lot because I am the right person.

I can climb mountains.

I can reverse any reality.

I approve of everything I do.

All my decisions are taken in hindsight, and these are good for me.

I am unique.

I believe in myself inconsiderately.

I think positively.

Understanding is one of my most important qualities.

I have all the qualities in me to reach my ends.

I am determined to deal with all situations.

I am a man capable of exceeding my limits.

I am a unique person with great qualities.

I am the right person, and I deserve happiness.

All my decisions are good at different levels.

Serenity is an integral part of me.

Every day I weigh myself, the scales show significant weight loss.

Each day I successfully lose weight without fail.

My weight loss program is working like magic.

I have a happy and healthy attitude towards life.

I love my body; that is why I want the best for it.

My body is responding immensely to my weight loss efforts.

I can feel my body fats melting away.

I have developed a high rate of metabolism that helps me reach my ideal weight.

I have a complete focus on my weight loss journey.

When I set a goal, I make sure I achieve it.

Every day I wake up challenged and determined to reach my ideal weight goal.

No one and nothing can stop me from getting into the best shape of my life.

My determination to lose weight cannot be deterred.

My motivation to exercise is exceptional.

Every day I am motivated to follow a regular exercise regimen.

I am self-motivated and inspired to lose weight and follow a healthy lifestyle.

Being healthy is not only a lifestyle for me but a principle that I am determined to keep.

I choose to be a healthy and fit person.

I choose to eat healthily and maintain an active lifestyle.

I choose to feel fit and sexy.

My mind is hard-wired to want only healthy food, and my body automatically feels that need for daily physical activity.

My mind only accepts Positive thoughts and compliments about my body and resists any negativities that can divert me from my weight loss goal.

I am surrounded by people who help and motivate me during my weight loss journey.

I am worthy of good health.

I focus on positive progression.

I am a friend to my body.

I look after my body with unconditional compassion.

It feels good to exercise.

My metabolism is working to my advantage by helping me gain my optimal weight.

I am thankful for my body for all the things it does for me.

I know what to eat and how to live my life.

Every physical movement I make helps me maintain my ideal body weight.

The more I move, the better I feel.

My stomach is toned, my arms are toned I-am-in-shape.

I find it easy to stay in shape.

I'm grateful for my healthy, fit body.

I am in control of how the amount of food I eat.

Following a healthy eating plan is easy for me.

Eating healthy foods helps my body get all of the nutrients it needs to be in the best shape.

My metabolism is fast.

I acknowledge the beauty my body holds.

I believe in myself and acknowledge my greatness.

I bring the qualities of love into my heart.

I can accept myself for who I am.

Every day, I am getting closer to my ideal weight.

I am capable of achieving my goals.

I am happy about the feeling of wellness these changes are bringing me.

Every day, I increasingly love my body.

Trusting my body is becoming easier.

I stay focused on my ideal size.

This is my body; I treat it with respect and honor.

I am at peace with my body.

My body is being restored to its natural state of excellent health.

Love and affection flow into my life with ease.

I appreciate life.

All my wildest dreams and every good thing is flowing to me effortlessly and smoothly.

I'm entirely motivated to live a healthy life.

I have the power in me to make good things happen

I am becoming fitter and stronger every day through exercise.

I celebrate my power to make good and healthy choices around food.

I eat healthy meals.

Every day I am exercising and taking care of my body.

I am efficiently controlling my weight through a combination of healthy eating and exercising.

I maintain my ideal weight, and I enjoy life being fit.

I love the feeling exercising gives me.

I find time to exercise.

When I exercise, I feel powerful and alive.

I am burning calories every day.

I love exercising, and I love working out, I love eating natural foods.

It is easy for me to control my weight.

I love the taste of healthy food.

It's exciting to discover my unique food and exercise system for my ideal weight.

Everything I eat heals nourishes my body, and helps mc reach my ideal weight.

I have a strong urge to eat only healthy foods and to let go of any processed foods.

I only eat nutritious foods, and I can easily resist temptations.

I am so grateful now that I have healthy eating habits.

Eating healthy comes naturally to me.

Healthy, nutritious food is what I eat every day.

My body benefits from the healthy food that I eat.

Healing is happening in both my mind and heart.

Healing happens with each step I take.

I quickly reach and maintain my ideal weight

I do what it takes to be healthy.

Every day I am getting slimmer and healthier.

I am a beautiful person inside out.

I can truly love myself for who I am.

I am grateful for the body shape I have been blessed with.

I accept myself for who I am.

I am grateful for the body I have.

I am getting closer to my ideal weight every day.

I am losing weight because I want to and because I have the power to do this.

Making changes is natural to me.

I am healthier and stronger with each day that passes.

Today, I focus on the good things that are unfolding in my life.

Every day is a new beginning.

I love my beautiful body.

I am content, peaceful, and full-filled.

I lovingly allow love, joy, and good health to flow through my mind and my body.

I am loved and am loving.

I am grateful for life and my body.

I am peaceful, joyful, and centered.

I believe in myself, and I will succeed.

I often visualize myself in my ideal weight

Exercising is fun, and it makes me feel outstanding.

I am happily exercising every day

I eat fruits and vegetables daily

Exercising is fun.

I am the person I think I am.

I agree with the people around me and trust my colleagues.

Self-esteem is my paramount quality.

My life is plenty of confidence.

I am a confident person who keeps getting better every day.

I trust my choices, and I move in that direction.

I erase in my life all the people who prevent me from achieving happiness.

I control my choices and my life.

I am responsible for my positive mental state.

I deserve a fulfilling life.

What I feel is healthy.

Trust in me is my first quality.

I attract good in my life.

I will offer everything I have given.

Love is present; it is enough that I believe in it.

I am aware that my friends love me.

I have a family and relatives who surround me.

I have a fulfilling social life.

I am in love.

I make the world better every day.

I like family time.

I take the time necessary to show my entourage how important they are to me.

I love them.

I can take time for myself and my loved ones.

Compassion is part of me.

I can give forgiveness.

I practice benevolence with conviction to help my entourage to evolve.

I can question myself and understand.

I choose to do what I like.

I believe in love.

I let my heart speak.

I can let people love me.

I like others, and others love me in return.

I accept that others can love me.

Fusional / passional love is coming into my life.

The people I love me back.

I can give love to others.

If I give others love, they make it exponentially.

I can attract the person I want.

My sentimental relationships are healthy and fulfilling.

I'm ready to fall in love.

I give a lot because I love this person

Love is in me.

Love is only an extension of my fulfillment.

Joy filled me and filled my life.

The people around me are filled with love, and I benefit from it.

I'm falling in love.

The waves around me tell me that love is present.

Hidden love is real love.

I love to love a person.

I take the front and reveal my love.

As a magician, I chose to give love all around me.

I like people, even my enemies.

I receive love as I pass it.

My life is happy and joyful.

I feel good with this person.

My relationship is passionate, and I feel fulfilled.

I give everything to my companion to make her as happy as possible.

Love is an integral part of my life.

Passion paces my choices.

I can let my heart make decisions.

My heart is full of happiness.

Harmony is present in me.

I love life, and life loves me.

I understand my feelings and accept them.

I deserve to find love

I am endearing and open to others.

I can open myself to others.

I can confess the things that I feel.

I only feel positive things about the people around me.

I only transmit positive to those around me.

I focus on the things that make me happy.

I believe in the power of attraction.

I concentrate my efforts on what I want.

Money is a reward.

I can get as much money as I want.

Money is a form of remuneration that takes different forms, and I am already rich.

CHAPTER 18:

Love your body

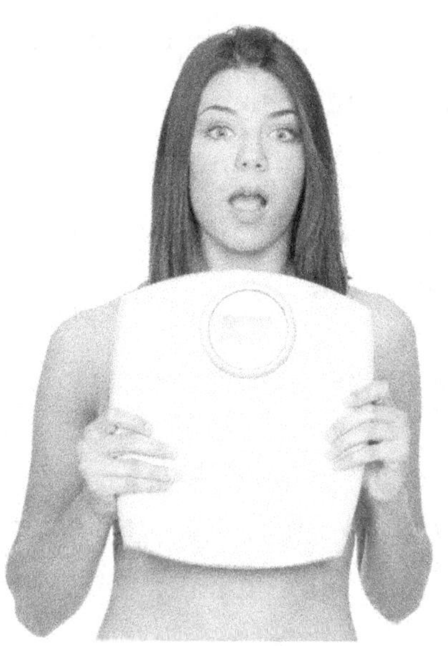

The majority of individuals don't think very much about self-improvement. We'd love to assist you in indulging in such a notion and finding out just how much you can enjoy yourself. It's a requirement to accept and create your ideal weight and everything else that's fantastic for you. Just being conscious of the idea of self-help can move you farther along on the way of enjoying yourself and accepting yourself as you are. Your character and character are aware of the way you're feeling on your own. If you harbor bitterness or remorse, or sense undeserving, these emotions operate contrary to enjoying yourself.

How can you see your flaws?

Can you blame yourself? Self-love and finding an error or depriving yourself repaint each other. It is tough to enjoy yourself if you frequently find errors ultimately.

Can you pay attention to the negative aspects of yourself?

Can you end up making self-deprecating statements, such as "I am not intelligent enough to..." or even "I am not great enough to..."?

Can you punish yourself or refuse yourself?

Can you establish boundaries with individuals who represent your very own moral and ethical criteria and your values and beliefs?

Look at the mirror. How do you feel about yourself? Can you smile or frown?

Which are you about the continuum of self?

Are you currently respectful and admiring?

Are you critical and judgmental, or would you love yourself for that you are?

Have you been cared for and caring for this individual who you see?

If you're ambivalent, then contemplate these concerns further. Be truthful with yourself. Have a conversation on your own. Take an honest look at yourself. Do not just examine your own body; examine your wisdom, your soul, your own emotions, along with your own heart. Know that: By enjoying yourself, you love yourself. If there's something that you can't accept on your own, be aware you could change that idea and alter it to make anything you want, such as your ideal weight.

How Does It Feel to Love Yourself?

Have a look at These features. Are these familiar to you? It is the way it should feel if you like yourself:

You genuinely feel happy and accepting your world, even though you might not agree with everything within it.

You're compassionate with your flaws or less-than-perfect behaviors, understanding that you're capable of improving and changing.

You mercifully love compliments and feel joyful inside.

You frankly see your flaws and softly accept them learn to alter them.

You accept all of the goodness that comes your way.

You honor the great qualities and the fantastic qualities of everybody around you.

You look at the mirror and smile (at least all the period).

Many confuse self-love with becoming arrogant and greedy. But some individuals are so caught up in themselves they make the tag of being egotistical and thinking just of these. However, we do not find that as a healthful self-indulgent character, which isn't well balanced in enjoying itself, love, and loving others.

It isn't selfish to get things your way; however, it's egotistical to insist that everybody else can see them your way. The Dalai Lama states, "If you do not enjoy yourself, then you can't love other people. You won't have the capacity to appreciate others. Suppose you don't have any empathy on your own. In that case, you aren't capable of developing empathy for others" Dr. Karl Menninger, a psychologist, states it this way: "Self-love isn't opposed to this love of different men and women. You can't truly enjoy yourself and get yourself a favor with no people a favor, and vice versa." We're referring to the healthiest type of self-indulgent, that simplifies the solution to accepting your best good.

Just take a better look at the way you see your flaws and blame yourself. Self-love and finding an error or depriving yourself aren't in any way compatible. If you deny enjoying yourself, you're in danger of paying too much focus on your flaws. That is self-loathing. You don't wish to focus on negative aspects of yourself, for by keeping these ideas in your mind, you're giving them the psychological energy which brings that result or leaves it actual.

Self-love is positive energy. Blame, criticism, and faultfinding are energy. Self-hypnosis can help you utilize your mind-body to make new and much more loving ideas and beliefs on your own. It helps your mind-body create and take fluctuations in the patterns of feeling and thinking that have been for you for quite a while, which aren't helpful for you. The trancework about the sound incorporates many positive suggestions to shift your ideas, emotions, and beliefs in alignment together with your ideal weight.

A Vital goal for all these positive hypnotic suggestions is the innermost feeling of enjoying yourself. If your self-loving feelings are constant with your ideal weight, it will likely occur with increased ease. But if you harbor bitterness or remorse, or sense undeserving, these emotions operate contrary to enjoying yourself enough to think and take your ideal weight. Lucille Ball stated it well: "Love yourself first and everything falls in line" The hypnotic suggestions about the sound are directions for change led to the maximum "internal" degree of mind-body or unconscious. However, the "outer" changes in life action should also happen.

Many weight reduction methods you have been using might appear to be a lot of work. We suggest that by adopting a mindset that's without the psychological pressure related to "needing to," "bad or good," or even "simple or difficult," with no judgment in any way, the fluctuations could be joyous.

Yes, even joyous. It produces the whole journey of earning adjustments and shifting easier. The term "a labor of love" implies you enjoy doing this so much it isn't labor or responsibility. The "labor" of organizing a family feast in a vacation season, volunteering at a hospital or school, or even buying a gift for someone very particular can appear effortless. Here is the mindset that will assist you in following some weight loss methods. We invite you to place yourself in the situation of being adored.

You're doing so to you. Loving yourself eliminates the job, which means it is possible to relish your advancement toward a lifestyle that encourages your ideal weight. Think about some action that you like to perform. Imagine yourself performing this action today. Notice that whenever you're doing something you love to perform, you're feeling energized and beautiful, and some other attempt is evidenced by enjoyment. At these times, you see it absolutely "loving what you're doing." Sometimes, we recommend that you also find that as "enjoying yourself doing this." Maybe by directing a more favorable attitude toward enjoying yourself, you'll end up enjoying what you're doing.

Giving Forth

Forgiveness is a significant step in enjoying yourself. At any time you forgive, you're "committing forth" or "letting go" of a thing you're holding inside you. Let's be clear about this: bias is simply for you, not anybody else. It's not a kind of accepting, condoning, or justifying somebody else's activities. It's a practice of letting go of an adverse impression that has remained within you too long. It's the letting go of any emotion or idea which can be an obstacle between you and enjoying yourself and getting what you desire.

A lot of us are considerably more crucial and much tougher on ourselves than others. When you continue to notions of what you should or should not have completed, you're not enjoying yourself. Instead, you're putting alert energy to negative beliefs about yourself. Ideas like "I should have obtained a stroll " or "I shouldn't have eaten this second slice of pie" can also be regarded as self-punishing. Sometimes, penalizing yourself, either by lack of overeating or eating, may even lead to a discount for your wellbeing. By shifting your focus to self-appreciation, you go from the negative to the positive, which is quite a bit more conducive to self-loving.

Writing in a diary about the wholesome choices you make every day may encourage self-improvement. By forgiving yourself and forgiving other people, you launch the psychological hold that previous events might have had on you, and you also make yourself accessible to appreciate yourself. When you launch the effects of earlier encounters by forgiving, you undergo reassurance and a calm comfort on your body, which helps you take your ideal weight.

You at the Head Table

Loving yourself involves placing yourself first. To drop fat and talk to the perfect weight of yours, you've to come. Therapist and writer Jean Fain wrote a post titled" The' Yes, I Will' Diet," originally printed in the 09/2005 issue of O: The Oprah Magazine. She recalls a forty-nine-year-old mum needed to drop pounds, telling her, "I do not care enough to care that I eat" She did not care about it in case she ate. She had not time for himself. Her life seemed to be in service that is constant to the demands of the husband of her, and the daughter of her, and her old mum, the company of her; they came. She ate junk food regardless of the weight reduction, taking blood pressure treatment, and the idea that a diet has been just a great deal, given her frame and plight of mind.

With her therapist's support, she found the time to hear relaxing CDs, find a massage, and see a book. Directly speaking, she discovered ways to put himself and tend to others with this high price itself. The article contained an email from twenty-five pounds lighter, saying, "I'm not at my goal yet, but I know that I shall succeed." Self-love and placing yourself go together. They're a winning combination. Any guilt you're feeling about putting yourself can be taken care of by fixing your reasons for feeling guilty and subsequently making decisions to eliminate them. Do anything is required to clean your path towards your ideal weight.

What Would You Like? What Do You Want?

Have you got a healthy self-image? There are lots of psychological tests that quantify self-image; however, our aim here isn't psychotherapy. So, let's just inquire, "Are you pleased with how you seem?" The question begs the following question: "What changes will please you?" There's no room for discretion, guilt, sorrow, or psychological energy to negative emotions. The questions and options are about what you'd like and exactly what you would like, followed by the ideas, beliefs, and activities that attract those outcomes around for you. Do you believe that your physical appearance influences how others treat you or feel about you?

Regrettably, the response for everybody is "yes." Body-size stereotypes are analyzed in many studies. Studies have shown that specialist therapists working with obese people have biases. If you're too heavy, you've felt that the others' prejudice throughout glances, ways of speech, and the differences in behavior toward you and the others of smaller size. Size-based discrimination could be hardest for children.

Along with the prejudice that kids have toward obese individuals is significantly rising. Research in 1961 reported that kids had discrimination against obese children. The study included revealing the kid's drawings and requesting them that they enjoyed the least. The four pictures portrayed kids, such as a kid in a wheelchair, yet a disfigured face, a person, known as "regular," and an obese kid. The drawing of this fat kid was chosen most frequently since the one that they enjoyed the least. This analysis was duplicated using 458 fifth-and sixth-grade kids in 2003.

In the new study, the difference between just how much they enjoyed the "ordinary" kid over the obese kid was greater than 40 percent higher than in 1961. Another study shows that adolescents who reported being teased about their weight have been dissatisfied with their bodies and considered attempted suicide. More Frequently than their peers who did not report being teased about weight.

These studies only validate that which any obese person perceives within our civilization. Overweight individuals don't require some reinforcement to dislike their self-image. The cultural and social biases and also body-size stereotypes produce debilitating feelings and might contribute to reducing self-esteem as well as weaker self-image. Evidently, at the social level, we will need to do a much better job of teaching ourselves about what's essential in valuing every individual and what's not. And we must approach problems of obesity using a more considerable sensitivity to individuals that weigh too much.

If you're experiencing difficulty with other people's glances and remarks about your body weight, use them to fuel your motivation to accomplish a wholesome body. Adopt the newest mindset, which each individual and each comment is presently a gift, not a curse. That's the way you should treat them as gifts. Each gift in the kind of an opinion about your weight is a reminder that you enjoy yourself, which you're moving toward your ideal weight, and that you're much more sensitive and compassionate than they are. Terry Cole-Whittaker composed a beautiful book titled Everything You Think of Me Is None of My Company. The publication title says everything and is a fantastic education about the best way best to

Conclusion

There are many reasons why someone should use hypnosis to lose weight. First, hypnosis is often successful when all other avenues of weight, health, and fitness have failed, and that's for a good reason!

The problem is not the method or even the plan you are using to achieve it. The problem is in your mind. If you want to lose real body fat, reduce weight, make your ideal shape, and maintain your new look, it is essential to change your attitude towards food and exercise and your behavior towards both.

The best hypnosis programs for weight loss may require you to understand and replicate those mental processes used by people who have lost weight already. It might be tough leaving your comfort zone. Hypnosis will help you reprogram your mind and install new thoughts that will become automatic habits once you identify the right behavior perfect for achieving your goal.

Eating less and adequately or exercise following a schedule won't be a dream anymore: hypnosis enhances and strengthens your will.

So, if you are worried about being overweight now, there is nothing wrong with undergoing hypnosis. After all, you have nothing to lose but weight.

Everything that comes from you that relates to you is just yours: your feelings, your voice, your actions, your ears, your thighs, your hopes, and your fears. That's why you are unique. Be happy that you are different from anyone, that you look the way you do and that it is just you. Start to feel that it's your own body, not something separate you need to live with.

Do you want your house to be just like anyone else's? Or do you love the little things that carry memories? Don't you love the atmosphere of your messy place after playing with your kids? And the plain curtain that you know you should replace, but which your mom sewed and looks so good? Or the piece of furniture that everyone says you should throw out, but you insist on it?

That's how you should feel about your body. You should understand that you don't need to compare it with anyone else's because it's impossible to compare unique things. Also, who determines what beautiful and ugly mean? You should not compare your body to the celebrities' perfect-looking bodies. First, because they are adjusted with Photoshop and other programs, and they are not real.

Ultimately, hypnosis, both in a professional or home setting, has the potential to help with weight loss. According to Vanderbilt University, hypnosis works best for individuals who need to lose low-to-moderate amounts of weight.

It doesn't mean that you shouldn't attempt it but talk with your doctor about working it into a routine that incorporates other weight loss behaviors. It requires a various number of hypnosis sessions by a hypnotherapist. It may take a long time before professional therapy alters your attitudes and actions, and it may take a while before changed behaviors become a habit.

Try not to get discouraged with little change. If nothing else, regular hypnosis sessions may help ease pressure and help you learn to relax, reducing your need to eat in emotional situations. Because hypnosis is probably not going to deal with the issue all by itself, consider keeping a food and exercise journal.

Also, record how long you practiced and what kind of activity you did. This log considers you accountable for poor decisions and allows you to distinguish patterns in your eating and exercise habits that may counteract healthy weight loss. When you identify these patterns, you'll have a venturing off point for your next hypnosis session, as far as critical thinking and behavior modifications may assist you with weight loss.

Regardless of how you approach hypnosis, its advantage may be what you have to finally lose that abundance of weight and carry on with a healthier life—good karma helps with using hypnosis to achieve your weight loss goals. Add up many small strides for weight loss success.

The more you practice the meditations we've given to you, the easier it will be to discover the success you've been waiting for. After a complicated diet, again and again, getting nowhere is an ideal opportunity to accept what isn't right about our mindset.

A perfect way to turn your mood around is to rework it through meditation. Tune in to these at whatever point you're home and find the opportunity. If you're exhausted, why not take a few minutes to relax and pull yourself together?

This meditation will be useful when you're feeling anxious. There may be a few evenings you may wake up and have trouble falling back asleep. Any one of these can help you relax while also encouraging you to fall into a weight loss mindset. Make sure you are placing yourself in a place where you can do these meditations safely.

Try not to drive with them, and regardless of whether you're taking a plane or other transportation where another person is in control, be cautious. When you do meditation, always do it at home in a safe place. Possibly, you will fall asleep without realizing it.

After you've attempted a few different reflections, you can use these methods on planes or anywhere else you may go if you know that you can stay awake and alert once you've come out of the meditation or hypnosis.

Recall that the meditations won't make you magically get more fit. They will help you get into the correct mindset necessary to finish the diet or exercise routine you are attempting. They will also assist you with relaxing and decreasing the pressure that can make this procedure harder.

Whatever strategy for eating healthy you may pick, these meditations and trances will help you stop gorging and think it is easier to eat healthily and practice naturally. Recollect that it takes over one attempt and that you should practice it regularly, not once a month. When you can incorporate these snapshots of relaxation into your routine, it will help them work better.

Good luck with your weight loss journey.